RETHINKING COMMUNICATION IN HEALTH AND SOCIAL CARE

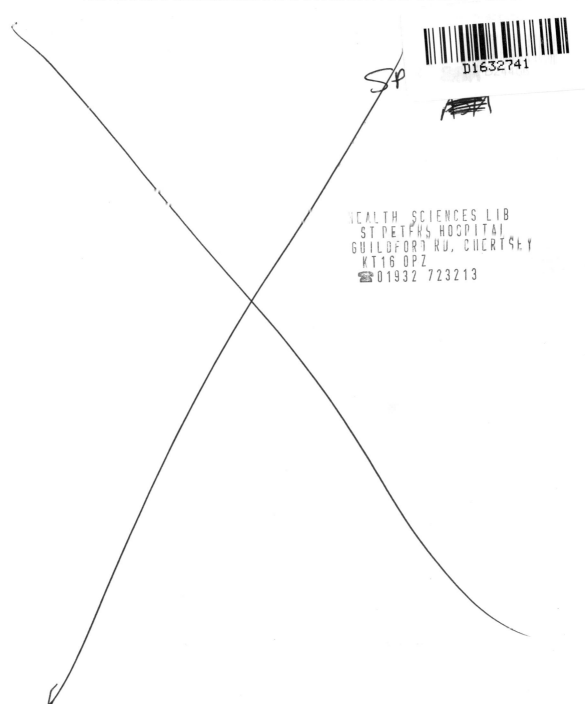

RETHINKING COMMUNICATION IN HEALTH AND SOCIAL CARE

ANNETTE ROEBUCK

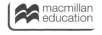 macmillan education   palgrave

LIST OF TABLES

QUOTATIONS

Guided Tour

The Key Features of Each Chapter in this Book Are:

Aims

By the end of this chapter you will be able to:

→ Identify different types of cultural groups to which you belong

→ Compare and contrast the different communication styles used in each of the groups

→ Assess the impact of differing cultural communication styles upon interpersonal exchanges

→ Describe how your cultural knowledge relating to vulnerable service users has developed

Each chapter begins with explicit Aims, to outline the topics you will be covering.

As Jeff left home this morning for his ballet practice he waved goodbye to his mother as he got into the taxi. It was his usual driver so he was able to just get in without saying anything and the car set off for the dance studio. During rehearsal he slipped and fell, banging his head. Since it was unclear whether he lost consciousness, he was taken to accident and emergency by one of the choreographers, Anne. Whilst in hospital, Anne was asked a lot of questions and Jeff was finding this irritating as no one was asking him, and he knew the answers. People were coming and going all the time and he wanted to go home. When he tried to get up to leave, people got cross and he was worried by this. He had to get home by 4pm because it was his day for going bowling with his friend Bob who relies on him to buy the tickets. He tried to explain that he had to leave, but when he said this, people weren't making any sense when they talked back to him. Whilst Anne went to the toilet, he wanted to try to explain again. As most of the staff looked cross, he wanted to find the smiley person with the white dress who didn't look scary. He thought her name was Sarah. When he did find her, she looked cross too. He was really confused by this.

Box 1.3: Case Scenario: Jeff

Case scenarios appear throughout to help you apply what you have learned to everyday practice.

Resource contents and tips for use

Chapter 4 Box 4.4 Audio link: I love you 	The words 'I love you' are spoken with differing types of pitch and emphasis to transmit the message in a variety of emotional tones. The exercise is designed to help you understand how changing the stress on words can totally change the emotional message that is received: even if there are only three words involved.

Chapter 5 Box 5.6
Space Invaders of the Intercultural Kind
  - A conference
  - A social gathering
 	
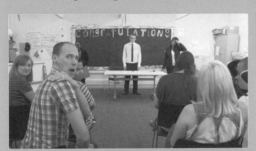
	Communicate2U show you how space can be used in different types of cultural settings.
	
	Conference
	The film based around the conference shows people filling up the seats at a conference venue. People who know each other well come in together in close proximity. They try to sit next to each other and as far away from strangers as the environment allows. As the room becomes more crowded, people are forced to sit next to one another. They tuck in their arms and legs so as to preserve as much personal space as possible and to minimise the risk of invasion into intimate space.
	
	People with a physical disability have limited options as to how to use social space in this setting as their area is pre-ascribed.
	
	The powerful speaker has their space pre-ascribed also, but they have the power to maintain a social distance from the less powerful audience.
	
	The Social Setting
	The after conference party shows two people from different national/ethnic backgrounds interacting. One prefers a closer personal distance to the other. Watch the discomfort of the previously powerful speaker as he is unconsciously chased into a corner!

Resource contents and tips for use

Chapter 5 Box 5.8
Learn From Us!

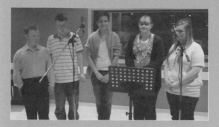

The word 'bay' in this song refers to both a hospital bay (the meaning that staff will have intended), and a seaside bay (the meaning picked up by service users).

The Makaton symbols shown are in a variety of 'dialects' – each person may perform these in a slightly different way. They include key things that staff need to recognise:

I want:
- My mum
- My dad
- The toilet
- Food (something to eat)
- Drink

I'm in pain

I want:
- A nurse
- A doctor
- Time to think

Communicate2U teach you the basic principles of communication in a song. The song includes the use of emblems in the form of Makaton as well as aspects covered in a number of earlier chapters such as:

- Looking at the person and talking to them
- Adjusting your pace of speech to a slower one
- Using simple words
- Remembering that simple words can have more than one meaning
- Remembering that people may have skills in lots of different areas. Just because they find words hard does not mean they don't have talents.
- Staff need to learn from the experts – US!

Chapter 6 Box 6.7
An Ordinary Ward Round?

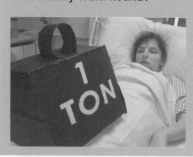

This short humorous piece shows how seemingly ordinary things (such as a tapping pen, a strong deodorant or flickering lights) can impact upon someone who is sensitive to this type of environmental input.

(Continued)

Resource contents and tips for use

Chapter 7 Box 7.7 **Mind Your Manners** 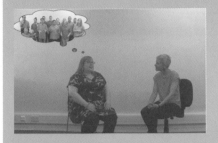	These two short films show a seemingly ordinary interaction between a professional and service user. Watch the speech bubbles to see what the service user is really thinking as the professional does their job ...
Chapter 7 Box 7.9 *Sea of Words* – **Ballet** 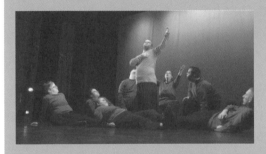	*Sea of Words* is a ballet performed by people with a learning disability who have very few words but excellent skills at communicating the emotional message through dance. Other pieces on the website transmit the message about how to communicate through song or drama. The use of dance here illustrates a form of communication that requires no words at all. The use of music, lighting, movement and space all combine to convey a strong message about how disempowering medical settings can feel. It could equally apply to a social care setting.
Chapter 7 Box 7.9 **You Talk to your Dog** 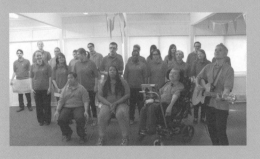	This song summarises the issues presented in this book and suggests a new script for staff to follow when interacting with vulnerable people. It argues that whilst staff may talk to their pets or shout at their computer and not be concerned that they cannot talk back, they often do not try to communicate well with people who are non-verbal. The song shows how vulnerable people feel when they are overlooked in communication exchanges. Communicate2U also teach you how to change the way that you communicate to make your interactions accessible.

CULTURE AND COMMUNICATION

Aims

By the end of this chapter you will be able to:

➡ Identify different types of cultural groups to which you belong

➡ Compare and contrast the different communication styles used in each of the groups

➡ Assess the impact of differing cultural communication styles upon interpersonal exchanges

➡ Describe how your cultural knowledge relating to vulnerable service users has developed

INTRODUCTION

At its heart, this book argues that all humans communicate. We can't help it. We feel something, whether it's a basic urge such as hunger, joy or pain, or a more complex one such as the desire to tell the world about an idea that is really important. We respond to that urge, and the result is communication. The form of communication may be relatively complex such as a book, or it may be as simple as the sound of a rumbling stomach, a smile or a wince. The result is still a message that is passed to people who are open to see or hear it. That brings us to the other central theme of this book: not everyone who works in health and social care settings is good at noticing simple communication. This is a problem, because the people who often need the most support, such as people with a learning disability (Goldbart *et al.*, 2010), dementia (DHHS, 2014; Gray *et al.*, 2007), mental health needs (DoH, 2011) or significant neurological impairment such as cerebral palsy (Balandin *et al.*, 2007b) may find it difficult or impossible to use the sophisticated skills that are associated with spoken communication. Even if people can use words, they may do so in a way that health and social care staff find alien. For example, the words may be foreign, produced by a voice commun-ication aid, or they may be in another format entirely such as a signed language. If people who work in health and social care settings are poor at recognising and responding appropriately to simple forms of communication, then they make people who rely upon this vulnerable. If you're reading this and thinking something along the lines of 'that's easy – I'm great at noticing simple messages' then you're off to a good start, and you may well be right. However, it's unlikely that you would have the words to effectively explain to other staff in health or social care settings why what you are doing seems to work for vulnerable people, and what may be occurring in their organisation that may prevent others from being as effective as you. It's also worth bearing in mind that many of the staff who have actively but inadvertently contributed to the pain and suffering of vulnerable people probably thought exactly the same thing. In the UK, poor staff communication with vulnerable service users is repeatedly highlighted as a significant factor in poor care or even avoidable deaths (Francis, 2013; Heslop *et al.*, 2013; Mencap, 2013; Mencap, 2006). The problem is often that every time that we communicate, we do so in a way that reflects the values and communication styles of one of the groups to which we belong. Groups can be as small as families or as big as organisations, professional groups or nations. However, once we're in those groups it's very difficult for us to actually recognise our communication styles and we often fail to notice when we communicate badly with people whose style of interacting is different to our own (Hall, 1959; Scollon *et al.*, 2012). This chapter will help you to understand the different groups that you belong to and the different styles of communication that they adopt. It will compare your styles of communication with those of vulnerable people and support you to use that knowledge to understand the difficulties that can occur when people from different groups come together. It will do so by considering those groups as cultures.

DEFINING CULTURE

Culture is difficult to define, not only because it means different things to different people, but also because as soon as you group things into one category, you run the risk of excluding them from another. For example, you may consider a trip to the ballet to be a cultural experience, but it is unlikely that an intercultural theorist would frame culture in this way. In its broadest sense, culture encompasses concepts such as the values that groups of people hold, the sets of rules that people have to follow if they want to be accepted within the group, and the things that they do to actively enact those principles (Scollon *et al.*, 2012). Common to most definitions of culture is the idea that groups develop norms for interactions, but those norms are implicit and often hidden from the group members themselves (Bowe *et al.*, 2007; Jandt, 2007). Communication is complex, and to manage the mass of information, cultural communication theorists may focus upon specific aspects such as spoken and written language forms (Bowe *et al.*, 2007) or the use of time and space (Hall, 1977; Hall, 1959; Mehrabian, 1971) to give just a couple of examples. This book is particularly concerned with theorists who have explored aspects of culture that are generally hard to see, such as differences in how the use of time and personal space are viewed (Hall, 1977; 1959) or how we respond to interactions with people who seem not to be communicating with us at all (Watzlawick, 1978; Watzlawick *et al.*, 2010). It is also concerned with how health and social care professionals consciously or unconsciously manage their image (Goffman, 1967; Goffman, 1959), particularly when interacting with service users and families who fall outside of societal norms (Goffman, 1968; Goffman, 1961; Goffman, 1963). This book therefore predominantly focuses upon what people do within face to face interactions and draws upon the idea that culture is actually a verb – something that is 'done' and not just an abstract concept (Scollon et al., 2012). Therefore, culture is defined as the normative patterns of behaviour and communication developed over time and enacted by people who share, or are affected by, common values and beliefs. The term 'intercultural communication' is a term that will be used within the book to explore the face to face interactions between people from different cultural backgrounds (Jandt, 2007:7).

Before we start to explore cultural communication in more depth, you need to first recognise that this is something that you are already doing. Have a go at the exercise in Box 1.1 to explore the ways in which you already adapt your communication to meet the expectations of different communication partners.

> ## Different settings, different communication styles
>
> 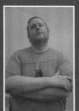 Think of all the people you remember interacting with on one fairly busy day last week. Include people who served you in shops, colleagues or tutors, family and friends. Think about how you spoke to each one.
>
> **?** **Did you communicate the same way in each situation?**
>
> **?** **How did your communication differ?**
>
> **Box 1.1:** Communicating in different settings

 ## CULTURAL LENSES

When we think of culture we often think of people who come from a different country, or who have a different ethnic background to our own. The potential impact of cultural misunderstandings between people with these types of differences is increasingly being recognised in health and social care literature (for examples see Comas-Diaz, 2012; Kidd, 2010; Laird, 2008; Raghavan, 2009). Whilst this chapter will touch briefly on some of these aspects, it will not be the main focus. Instead we will be exploring the more mundane and hidden aspects of culture that arise because we are members of a particular family, social group or profession. These day to day interactions can be so routine that we never even consider them as being culture at all, yet they have the potential to impact upon vulnerable service users to the point that they can jeopardise health and well-being. Life is so complex that we have to select what to focus upon, so each of us will pay attention to different aspects of a situation. The way in which we do this will be influenced by the experiences of previous generations who have passed their knowledge down to us, as well as our own life experiences. The result of so many influences is that we can end up holding quite complex and conflicting ideas; we can hold many different attitudes towards the same thing at the same time. For example, as a health or social care professional it is hoped that you would never think of calling someone with a learning disability an idiot: you know that this is a form of abuse and it would be unprofessional to do so. Yet, by the same token you may well use that word, or one very similar to it when you shout at a driver who has narrowly missed hitting you. By using that term in that way you are enacting a deeply embedded societal view of people who have reduced intellectual capacity since words such as 'idiot', 'moron' and so on are historical terms for this client group. The words are never used in a positive way – they are used to indicate people you deem to have lesser value. They are words you will have learned in the playground or within your family, and you carry that hidden knowledge with you every time you enter your work setting, even if you overlay it with professional knowledge.

Understanding the hidden cultural knowledge within you is crucial if you are going to be an effective communicator with vulnerable people. Culture is multifaceted, and to help you understand some of the concepts that are presented, they will be explored by using the analogy of lenses. In photography or in science, different lenses can be used to filter out some information to allow the viewer to focus on important items in more depth. The object can be seen through many different lenses – the object remains the same, but the way that it is viewed alters. The lenses within this chapter are designed to help you to identify how you may frame your interactions with others with reference to the different cultural groups to which you belong. The case scenarios below will be used during the chapter to illustrate how culture and communication affect the way in which we interact with one another in different settings. You get quite a bit of information on Sarah within this case scenario, and in case you feel that David is being treated unfairly, please note that you will get more information on him towards the end of this chapter.

Sarah is a nurse who works in a busy accident and emergency unit in an inner city hospital in England. She is conscientious and cares deeply for those people in her care. Before leaving home today she kissed her partner Joe goodbye, and waved to her neighbour. During her shift she worked with colleagues from a wide variety of disciplines; doctors, volunteers, therapists, paramedics, managers, cleaners and support staff. The patients that she met reflected the diverse ethnic population of the city and ranged in age from babies to the very elderly. Today was particularly trying as she had a couple of patients who were told to go to their cubicles, but they kept wandering into other areas, causing havoc. To help unwind, she chatted to her friend David, who is a social worker who specialises in supporting families where a member has severe dementia. He experiences similar problems and feelings. David had also had a rough day as a client he was particularly close to had wandered away from his accommodation, triggering safeguarding concerns that he was asked to address. Sharing these experiences helped both of them to get some perspective. David was going to go to the gym to relax before he went home. Sarah listened to music on the radio on the way home as well to help relax, because she knew that Joe had a stressful meeting today. If they talked about work when they were tired they would end up bickering. Joe was really tired and despite her good intentions they had an argument about who was going to cook. Although he didn't say so, she knew he was sorry because he brought her a glass of wine as they watched the soap opera together. Sarah sometimes misses some of the storylines because of her shift patterns, so keeping up with the plot can be a challenge during the week. Trying to watch the omnibus edition at the weekend is a nightmare because her mum comes around for dinner and is forever interrupting the viewing by asking questions about what's happening! She doesn't want to offend her mum though and tries to hide her irritation. She talks about this with her friends at the hockey club when she plays at the weekend.

Box 1.2: Case Scenario: Sarah and David

When interacting with people from different disciplines, ethnic backgrounds, ages and who have different types of personal relationships with her, Sarah will have adapted her communication style. As a nurse, her job is important to her so she will act in accordance with her professional values and training, striving to be caring and compassionate with all of her patients. She will also have used communication skills to understand the music that she listened to and the shows that she watched on TV. For the majority of the time, she will not have been consciously aware of doing this; she is only likely to have noticed communication issues when they became problematic to her, such as when the patients didn't do as they were asked. Even then, she may find it difficult to articulate exactly what has gone wrong, or why something seemingly so small such as her mum asking her a question as she watches TV can make her so frustrated. Sarah belongs to many different groups of people with whom she interacts on a regular basis. From a cultural perspective, these include her national identity as a citizen of the United Kingdom, her ethnic identity as a Scottish person working in England, her professional identity as a nurse, her identity as a member of a work organisation (the hospital), her family identity and her identity as a member of a social organisation (hockey club). These identities will be viewed as cultures later in this chapter. In the following scenario, try to identify some of the cultural groupings that Jeff belongs to.

As Jeff left home this morning for his ballet practice he waved goodbye to his mother as he got into the taxi. It was his usual driver so he was able to just get in without saying anything and the car set off for the dance studio. During rehearsal he slipped and fell, banging his head. Since it was unclear whether he lost consciousness, he was taken to accident and emergency by one of the choreographers, Anne. Whilst in hospital, Anne was asked a lot of questions and Jeff was finding this irritating as no one was asking him, and he knew the answers. People were coming and going all the time and he wanted to go home. When he tried to get up to leave, people got cross and he was worried by this. He had to get home by 4pm because it was his day for going bowling with his friend Bob who relies on him to buy the tickets. He tried to explain that he had to leave, but when he said this, people weren't making any sense when they talked back to him. Whilst Anne went to the toilet, he wanted to try to explain again. As most of the staff looked cross, he wanted to find the smiley person with the white dress who didn't look scary. He thought her name was Sarah. When he did find her, she looked cross too. He was really confused by this.

Box 1.3: Case Scenario: Jeff

As well as being a son, ballet dancer, friend and bowler (which you may have easily spotted), Jeff also has a label of mild learning disability. The cultural groups to which he belongs have specific ways of communicating, just as Sarah's cultural groups did. Jeff often finds using words hard, but is very skilled at picking up on people's facial expressions and tone of voice. Over the years he's found ways of hiding the fact that he can't understand something. He helps support his friend Bob who finds using words in public even more difficult because of his stammer. He frequently experiences problems when interacting with people who use a lot of words, but has no problems at all at the ballet studios. There he's developed good friendships over the years and gets along with most people very well. Dancers don't tend to talk much whilst rehearsing – they may speak in short sentences, show each other how to improve a bit of technique, then get on with their rehearsal. This suits Jeff's communication style. He found it very irritating to be ignored whilst he was in the hospital as he is capable of answering the kind of questions that Anne was being asked and he was keen to show Anne that he could be in control of his hospital experience. Sarah was unaware that she had caused any distress during the day; she felt she had been professional and managed some crises effectively.

One of the biggest cultural barriers that Sarah faces is that she unconsciously measures her communicative effectiveness against the norms with which she is familiar. However, she would be hard pressed to articulate what those norms are in each of the roles that she occupies. When she encounters someone who has different norms, she doesn't have the tools to recognise ineffective communication and so fails to see the need to adapt her communication style. She is very unlikely to hear any complaints from people like Jeff because he finds words hard, lacks the confidence to speak up in the intimidating environment of the hospital and can't read the leaflets about how to make a complaint. Therefore, she continues to make the same mistakes. Her friend David, the social worker, is in exactly the same position. As a health or social care professional, you will also face the same challenges. Unless you can identify what your cultural norms of communication are and the impact that these may have on others with different norms, you run the very real risk of blindly going through your career hurting vulnerable people. As we will see later in the chapter, once you get into a position of authority, you may get to share your norms with others, so you also run the risk of passing these mistakes onto the next generation of professional staff, thus perpetuating the cycle of poor care for the most vulnerable communicators. The sections that follow are designed to help to reduce the risk of that occurring.

DIMENSIONS OF CULTURAL COMMUNICATION

Cultural communication norms can be considered as patterns of communication behaviours that have been internalised to such an extent that they are hidden from the people who enact them (Hall, 1959; Scollon et al., 2012). However, once those patterns are given names, it's much easier to understand what they are and to spot them. This section will give you the words you need to do this.

It's no wonder that patterns can become hidden as some of them may be very old indeed. For example it is argued that there are fundamental differences in the way that Western and Eastern cultures think and communicate and that these differences date back to the time of Aristotle in the West (circa 384 B.C.) and Confucius in the East (circa 551 B.C.). If you are from a Western culture such as that of Europe or North America, culturally speaking you are likely to view communication as consisting of a speaker who has an audience who receives the message. The roles may be reversed during the exchange, but the main purpose of speaking is to get a clear message to the other person. If you are from an Eastern background, such as that present in Japan, communication may primarily be viewed within the context of maintaining or strengthening relationships between members of the culture. The emphasis here is on selflessness, duty and a respect for hierarchy: the message itself is secondary to these goals (Jandt, 2007). The Western communicator wants a clear, concise answer to a question and finds the Eastern communicator to be evasive; the Eastern communicator finds the Western communicator to be abrupt and rude. Unhappiness and disharmony abound when people from the two cultures meet (Hofstede, 1994; Hofstede, 2001; Samovar *et al.*, 2004; Tong *et al.*, 2006). Cultural communication theorists can help to make the hidden patterns explicit to reduce the risk of poor communication occurring (Jandt, 2007). The East/West divide is of course somewhat simplistic. People will come from backgrounds that don't easily fit into these categories. Whilst the patterns reflect the ancient and fundamental divergence of East and West thinking by having two extremes, the diversity of communication styles that has developed over the intervening years is acknowledged by viewing the patterns as being on a spectrum. Seven dimensions of cultural communication on this spectrum that have been identified by key intercultural theorists (Hall, 1959; Hofstede, 1997; Hofstede *et al.*, 1984; Jandt, 2007; Neuliep, 2009) are presented for you to consider below:

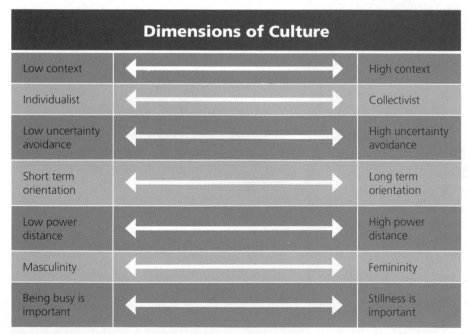

Dimensions of Culture

Low context		High context
Individualist		Collectivist
Low uncertainty avoidance		High uncertainty avoidance
Short term orientation		Long term orientation
Low power distance		High power distance
Masculinity		Femininity
Being busy is important		Stillness is important

Figure 1.1: Dimensions of cultural communication

You will be given a brief introduction to the key concepts associated with each of these dimensions, and the examples used will relate back to the case scenarios presented above in Boxes 1.2 and 1.3. You will be asked to undertake a few exercises and these are located within the boxes. Having gained a feel for the dimensions along which you communicate, you will then be introduced to some of the key cultural groups to which you belong and asked to relate these dimensions to your own cultures and communication styles.

Low and High Context Cultures

Hall's (1959) landmark book 'The Silent Language' introduced the idea that cultures differ according to how heavily interpersonal exchanges rely upon explicit communication (spelling out information, predominantly by using words) and how much is dependent upon implicit background knowledge.

Low context cultures value words to deliver a clear, detailed message. Since people in this type of culture do not share explicit knowledge of how to act in relation to one another, words are used to convey information clearly (Samovar et al., 2004). The topic under discussion is generally clearly and explicitly referred to early in the exchange. Communication within Western cultures such as the United Kingdom (UK) and the United States (US) generally follows this orientation (Hall, 1959; Scollon et al., 2012). This style of communication can also be seen within the context of organisational culture. Low context organisational cultures value commitment, privacy and adherence to the agreed plan (Jandt, 2007). Sarah's hospital work environment and David's social work environment could be classified as low context: both are expected to use words to transmit complex information accurately, and to ensure that protocols are strictly adhered to. National and local policies require them to record interventions in written and verbal formats, ensuring that other professionals within the team have access to this information whilst maintaining the principles of confidentiality. Both Sarah and David know that a failure to adhere to protocols carries strict penalties. That can make it feel difficult to acknowledge when something has gone wrong.

Within **high context cultures**, words are relatively unimportant compared to the context in which the communication occurs. What is important is the relationship between the communicators – their relative status, and expected role within the exchange (Hall, 1959). Such cultures emphasise group harmony and preserving relationships. When two people from the same high context culture meet, there is a shared understanding of values and patterns of communicating. The topic for discussion will generally not be specifically outlined,

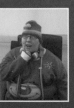

At a get together that includes family and friends, Pippa is asked where she went shopping. As she replies 'Shrewsbury' she glances across to her mother who starts laughing. Pippa then joins in the laughter. Others in the group look a little confused but continue the conversation. Pippa and her mother know that she struggles to pronounce the name of the town, and it has become an in-joke within the family.

Think about your own family or close friendship groups.

? **Are there similar examples of in-jokes?**

? **Would a stranger to the group understand the joke without an explanation?**

Box 1.4: High context communication within families

but alluded to, knowing that the other person shares the background knowledge (Samovar *et al.*, 2004). In this respect, families often have the characteristics of a high context culture (Hall, 1959) as a shared history may mean that the context of a situation makes words relatively redundant as the example in Box 1.4 illustrates. A high context organisation values the people within the organisation and works to foster relationships between workers. There is flexibility, friendliness and openness (Jandt, 2007). Jeff's ballet troupe is linked to a national ballet company and the dancers all have a label of learning disability. Communication within his sessions can also be classed as high context as everyone knows people's individual communication styles well, and they adapt to one another easily. Words are rarely used as gestures or demonstrations are more effective. When things go wrong, people are usually open about the problem and work together to solve it.

As with all subsequent sections that relate to cultural dimensions, you are advised to consider these as cultural tendencies, rather than absolute states. David knows that whilst a client walking off a unit without being noticed shows that there is a problem, he also knows that his manager will be keen to understand not only potential breaches in protocols, but also other contextual factors that may have led to the problem. The choreographers in Jeff's ballet troupe sometimes get involved in technical discussions in front of the dancers, forgetting that their words may not be understood by the people with a learning disability. Cultures may exhibit a mix of characteristics and the summary of the spectrum shown below needs to be considered within this context.

Figure 1.2: Summary of the communication characteristics of low and high context cultures

Individualism and Collectivism

Individualism and collectivism are terms that refer to how important the needs of the individual are in relation to that of the group (Hofstede, 1994; 1997).

In an **individualist** culture, as the name suggests, the individual and their immediate family are of primary importance. Goals are set according to the priorities of the person and their family first, with other parties having minimal priority (Jandt, 2007). In order to achieve these goals in a culture where others

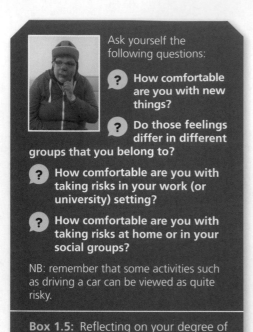

Ask yourself the following questions:

? How comfortable are you with new things?

? Do those feelings differ in different groups that you belong to?

? How comfortable are you with taking risks in your work (or university) setting?

? How comfortable are you with taking risks at home or in your social groups?

NB: remember that some activities such as driving a car can be viewed as quite risky.

Box 1.5: Reflecting on your degree of comfort with risk and uncertainty

are also striving to have their needs prioritised, there has to be a degree of competition between individuals. The United States is an example of a highly individualist culture where what people have achieved and how much success they have is seen as a measure of their value. American values have been postulated as being based on individual self-interest, self-gratification and independence and the government exists for the benefit of the individual (Hsu, 1969). Sarah and David come from the UK, which also tends towards an individualist outlook: their families are the most important thing in their lives, and their individual achievements are important to them.

In a **collectivist** culture the emphasis is on relationships between people, and individual needs may be subsumed into a goal that benefits wider society. Harmony amongst people is an important goal, and who you are related to is more important than individual success. For example, Chinese value systems are identified as filial duty and respect for elders, hard work, harmony and observing social rituals (Chinese Cultural Connection, 1987). Whilst neither David nor Sarah identify with these values in their private lives, they both work in professions and organisations that have some features seen in collectivist cultures. Sarah works in the National Health Service, which works with individuals in need but is also an organisation dedicated to benefitting society as a whole (NHS, 2015a). As a social worker, David is committed to the values of social justice and supporting oppressed individuals, but with a view to also shaping society to improve the lives of marginalised societal groups (Hepworth *et al.*, 2009; Reamer, 2013).

Figure 1.3: Summary of the communication characteristics of individualist and collectivist cultures

Low Uncertainty Avoidance – High Uncertainty Avoidance

Uncertainty avoidance is the degree to which members of a culture feel threatened by new or unknown things. **Low uncertainty avoidance** cultures tend to be more relaxed and are relatively comfortable with taking risks. People tend to be contemplative in outlook (Jandt, 2007). Whilst the members of Jeff's ballet company who have a learning disability often feel threatened by the unknown in other aspects of their lives, the ballet company where they work has a low uncertainty avoidance tendency and they feel safe. Setting up this type of company was a risk, and for sessions to work there has to be a relaxed attitude to the unexpected occurring. David's manager is working to create a similar ethos in the social work team: whilst risks have to be carefully weighed and managed, the nature of dementia means that if clients are to maintain some quality of life, risks have to be taken. David encounters the unexpected on a daily basis and feels relatively comfortable with this.

High uncertainty avoidance cultures tend towards security-seeking acts that may have a more aggressive tone, and members can be emotional and intolerant (Jandt, 2007). Each time change occurs, staff tend to feel threatened and uncomfortable. Sarah's hospital workplace tends towards high uncertainty avoidance. There are numerous policies and procedures in place to reduce the risk of things going wrong, and people who make mistakes are formally held to account. Risks are to be eliminated wherever possible. Sometimes there are strongly worded discussions amongst the team. Some professionals feel that patients need to take some risks in order to be prepared for life at home, and other professionals feel that they should take no risks in the hospital setting as the hospital may then be open to complaint and litigation.

Figure 1.4: Summary of the communication characteristics of low and high uncertainty avoidance cultures

Long Term Time Orientation – Short Term Time Orientation

Time orientation refers to how important past and future events are to current interactions, and the length of time over which the culture is prepared to work for a purpose. **Long term orientation** cultures tend to be those that emphasise working towards a common goal for the good of all. Many Eastern cultures have this view (Jandt, 2007). Perseverance and thrift are important factors in achieving this, so individuals may have to go without today so that society as a whole can benefit in the future. Time may be considered in terms of generations, rather than an individual's life span. Coming from the UK, Sarah and David sometimes struggle to understand families who are prepared to wait for generations for change to occur as they are working to create change that will benefit their individual clients during their life span.

The United States, Australia, New Zealand, Great Britain and Pakistan are examples of cultures that tend towards a **short term orientation** in which quick results are preferred, and people are prepared to spend money now to achieve this (Hofstede, 2001). Sarah and David both work in organisations that have a short term orientation, and their home life too reflects this perspective. Although Jeff works in an organisation with this perspective, he has a very limited concept of time, and sometimes struggles when he has appointments with people who are driven by the clock.

Figure 1.5: Summary of the cultural characteristics of long and short term time orientations

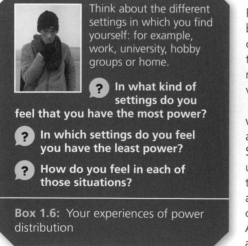

Think about the different settings in which you find yourself: for example, work, university, hobby groups or home.

? In what kind of settings do you feel that you have the most power?

? In which settings do you feel you have the least power?

? How do you feel in each of those situations?

Box 1.6: Your experiences of power distribution

High Power Distance – Low Power Distance

Power has an intrinsic link with communication and because of this it is explored in depth in the next chapter (Chapter 2). Here, we introduce the idea that whenever power exists, some people will hold more than others, and the way that it is distributed varies in different cultures (Hofstede, 1997).

When there is a **high power difference**, wealth, prestige and power are concentrated in a small number of individuals (Hofstede, 2001). Superiors and subordinates expect to have unequal access to power processes, and nations that exhibit these tendencies tend to be more authoritarian in outlook. At a family level, children are expected to show deference to elders. At an organisational level, there is a hierarchical approach to accessing decision-making processes and power, with those at the bottom of the organisation having limited access to those at the top (Jandt, 2007). Sarah feels that as a nurse, whilst she has some power over her immediate workspace, within the National Health Service as a whole, she is relatively powerless, despite the introduction of policies that are designed to be empowering (Currie *et al.*, 2015). She feels that politicians dictate policies that she is subject to, and managers control her departmental priorities. She knows she has limited access to any real power to make a difference. Whilst meetings are held to discuss departmental issues, managers control the agenda and expect their concerns to take priority. Her organisation could be considered to have a high power difference.

Cultures with a **low power difference** distribute power more evenly amongst the population. People tend to treat each other more as equals (Hofstede, 2001). Within low power difference organisations, subordinates would expect to be consulted and their ideas to be valued within decision-making processes. Managers would play a minimal role during disagreements, relying on peers to help to resolve conflict (Tyler *et al.*, 2000). The organisations in which both Jeff and David work can be described as having lower power difference tendencies. There is an expectation that workforce and managers will negotiate workload and priorities. Jeff gets to decide some of his own dance moves, and can help select which performances the troupe will attend. David and his manager work together to resolve difficulties. In their home lives, Sarah, Jeff and David all experience low power difference cultures – all family members can influence decisions. All three have grown up in the United Kingdom, which is a low power country (Hofstede, 2001), and their families reflect Hofstede's (1997) belief that power difference tendencies are learned early in childhood within family settings that reflect the wider national approach to power.

Figure 1.6: Summary of the characteristics of high and low power difference cultures

Masculinity – Femininity

Masculinity/femininity cultural identity affects the ways in which people who are labelled male, female, gay, straight, cross gendered or any other word that is linked to these concepts, are expected to behave and communicate. Feminine traits are considered to include compassion and emotionality. Masculine traits include strength, assertion and competitiveness (Jandt, 2007). The degree to which countries and cultures are tolerant of role overlap occurring varies (Hofstede, 2001).

Sarah and David occupy work roles that require them to demonstrate the values of compassion and concern for the weak (NHS, 2015a; NHS, 2015b;

Reamer, 2013; Sheedy, 2013). These are traditionally associated with femininity, and UK culture generally is not very tolerant of role overlap (Hofstede, 2001). As a ballet dancer, Jeff also occupies a role that has a strong association with femininity. Sarah has not experienced any problems with others judging her choice of career. David and Jeff on the other hand sometimes get teased by others outside of the work setting for choosing roles that are 'girly'.

Figure 1.7: Summary of masculine and feminine traits

Activity and Stillness

The final dimension in this section relates to the types of activities that people undertake within a culture, and the perceived value that they hold. Some cultures view work and occupations as being activities that help to define us as human beings and reflect our overall worth. In these cultures it is important to be busy and to develop new skills. Western cultures often have this orientation. Eastern cultures on the other hand often view stillness and contemplation as being an important component of life. People from the West may view people from the East as being lazy, and conversely, people from the East may view those in the West as being impetuous (Jandt, 2007; Neuliep, 2009). Sarah and David both feel that it is important to work hard and can get impatient with colleagues who are not busy and who seem to be daydreaming. As they both have lots of hobbies, they privately feel that some of their friends are wasting their lives because they don't seem to do much outside of work. Jeff needs to take time to think things through and whilst he has many hobbies, is also happy to have some quieter time.

Figure 1.8: Summary of the characteristics of activity and stillness

Having viewed the patterns that make up cultures, we will now explore how those patterns develop.

LEARNING CULTURAL NORMS

By now you should have an idea as to the patterns of behaviour that influence the ways that Jeff, Sarah and David communicate in different cultural settings. When the dimensions are brought together they form **cultural norms** that encompass a whole range of taken for granted aspects of life. We tend to create patterns of knowledge based on what those around us perceive to be meaningful, and disregard knowledge that our societal group does not value (Hall, 1959). During our earliest months of life, we live in a world that is dominated by our senses.

We gradually learn to perceive and interpret what we see, hear, smell, touch, taste and feel (Ayres, 1979; Jandt, 2007), but as there is an overwhelming amount to take in, we are culturally sensitised to pick out what is important. Norms are therefore learned. For example, now that Sarah has a lot of experience she is generally very good at picking up cues that tell her what needs to be done within her busy hospital department. She knows and responds to the cultural norms. However, if she were to be transported to a jungle, she would find it very hard to pick out which of the many fast moving shadows is likely to be a dangerous animal as this is an alien culture to her. If you doubt the strength of this type of cultural programming, have a look at the classic study by Tonys and Chabris (1999) in which participants viewing a basketball game totally failed to notice unexpected visual stimuli that came onto the court during the match. The participants were culturally programmed to focus upon the quality of movements that resulted in scores or moved the game forward. The unusual stimuli that came into view included a woman with an umbrella going onto the court and a person in a gorilla costume that was in shot for five seconds! The study noted that this type of inattention is particularly common in busy environments. As a health or social care professional you will be spending much of your time at work in busy environments. Even clinical experts who are trained to look for abnormalities experience this phenomenon (Drew *et al.*, 2013). Experience does not make you immune to error: it may make you more prone to overlooking things that fall outside of your normal experience, just as

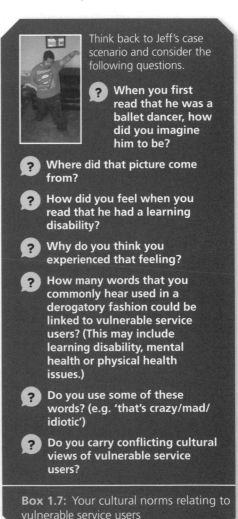

Think back to Jeff's case scenario and consider the following questions.

? When you first read that he was a ballet dancer, how did you imagine him to be?

? Where did that picture come from?

? How did you feel when you read that he had a learning disability?

? Why do you think you experienced that feeling?

? How many words that you commonly hear used in a derogatory fashion could be linked to vulnerable service users? (This may include learning disability, mental health or physical health issues.)

? Do you use some of these words? (e.g. 'that's crazy/mad/idiotic')

? Do you carry conflicting cultural views of vulnerable service users?

Box 1.7: Your cultural norms relating to vulnerable service users

Sarah did when she failed to notice her poor communication with Jeff. We naturally develop cultural norms, and they help us to manage the complexities of our environments. However, as the examples above illustrate, they carry with them the danger of cultural blindness.

Some of the most fundamental norms that we carry with us will have developed in childhood at a preconscious level (Berger *et al.*, 1969; Hall, 1959). These are then overlaid with knowledge that is consciously taught to us by others – for example, by parents, or professional educators with a legitimated role to pass on knowledge. Knowledge can be transmitted in three main ways, with varying degrees of emotional connection associated with each (Hall, 1959). Emotional connections are important as they determine how deeply we embed the knowledge that we have gained (Weiss, 2000).

1. **Informal learning** is principally based on the concept of modelling (Bandura, 1971). It occurs during childhood when we learn through observation without even realising that we are learning at all. The rules for the behaviours that we engage in are very well hidden. For example, when we learn how to climb a tree by watching others do the same. As long as things are progressing normally, there is little emotion associated with things that we learn informally. However, if these hidden norms of behaviour are breached, we are likely to feel very anxious without knowing why. Since informal knowledge is so hidden, it is pervasive, and it can be difficult to know what it is that needs changing. As children, both David and Sarah saw the slow kids being called names in the playground. They were called words like idiot, moron or nutcase. As adults they use these words as derogatory terms outside of the work setting without a second thought.

2. **Formal learning** is that which is taught by parental type figures using example and punishment – e.g. learning table manners by being shown how to sit up, and being told off for using the fork in the wrong hand. There are hundreds and hundreds of finely nuanced details to behaviour that are learned in this way. Over time these equate to a hidden formal system of behaviour: for example, we are polite to our elders; we don't interrupt. Since we learn this type of knowledge from parental figures, violations of formal norms are associated with strong emotions as they touch upon our childhood foundations. Sarah and David were both brought up by their parents to 'be nice' to other people and to take care of those who are struggling. Sarah had a friend who had a weird brother Gary who was a bit slow, and she often tried to make sure they didn't play with him. She felt guilty about this. Formal systems of knowledge are very resistant to change.

3. **Technical learning** is knowledge that is transmitted by members of the culture who have a specific role to pass information on, for example educators. This type of learning is done in an unemotional, logical way, with feelings suppressed since they interfere with efficient working. In their jobs, Sarah and David now have technical words that they can use to describe the people who are slow or weird: they have a learning disability or mental health problem. They would never call them an idiot, moron or nutcase. They have learned to put their emotions to one side when confronted by distressing

cases in order to function and fulfil their obligations to the client. Technical systems of knowledge that are not associated with strong emotions are the most superficial. Learning may not be deeply embedded, and therefore it can unconsciously be over ridden by informal or formal learning. However, lack of emotional investment also means that it is generally the easiest type of learning to change, providing change can be logically presented.

When Sarah was interacting with Jeff in the hospital, all three modes of learning affected her communication. As a child at school she absorbed the informal cultural norm that tell her that speed and intelligence are valued: people who are slow have lesser worth in exams, in the classroom and in the playground. The formal learning from her parents that told her she should be nice to everyone was at odds with her informal learning: she didn't like playing with Gary and tried to avoid it. As she was quite good at doing this she didn't ever learn a way of communicating effectively with him, or others like him. During her training she had a session on learning disability and learned about the communication deficits that this client group has, and how to overcome them. It was one session out of many and she has forgotten most of the details as she works on a general ward and this isn't her speciality. Her technical learning was not effective in overcoming the imbedded informal patterns that she experienced on a daily basis in the playground during her childhood. Neither she nor David saw any incongruence between their professional and private roles when using a word such as 'idiot' as a term of abuse outside of work. The usage is so deeply embedded within many of the settings that they experience that they have become blind to its deeper meaning. They fail to see that when they use that word they are enacting a cultural norm that links undesirable behaviours with people who have reduced intellectual capacity.

You may learn new cultural values and norms as you take on a professional role, but the ones that you learned in childhood don't simply disappear – they are still a part of you. Unless you can recognise these ingrained norms of behaviour and communication, they will impact upon your professional roles in ways that you don't even notice. The rest of this book is about helping you to recognise the deeply ingrained communication norms that you have in relation to people like Jeff and others who may generally be viewed as having lesser value by wider society. Technical (or academic) arguments support the views that are put forward to make it easier for you to make the changes in your behaviour. However, if you skip over the practical exercises that appear in the boxes, your learning will be superficial and you will not address the informal learning that shapes your interactions. You will make the same mistakes that Sarah made when she failed to notice that Jeff was communicating that he was worried and needed help.

Just like Sarah, David and Jeff, you inhabit many roles and are a part of many different cultures. The following sections are designed to help you understand the multiple cultural lenses through which you view life. This will prepare you to explore their impact on communication in health and social care settings in the chapters that follow. As you learn about each cultural lens, you will see an example as to how Sarah, David or Jeff are affected by the norms of that particular culture, and you will be asked to consider your own norms. At this stage you may find it difficult to articulate what some of those norms are as they are not only hidden, but may also be relatively abstract in nature. Therefore, you will need to do some work to help identify your cultural norms in a concrete way. Norms are often reflected in the values that we hold to be important, and the types of actions that we take that are in accordance with this value base. Exploring values is therefore the first step in this process.

Cultural values are beliefs that are held by pivotal members of that culture and by a majority of its members (Hofstede, 1994) but it can be very hard for us to actually identify what our cultural values are (Berger *et al.*, 1969; Hall, 1959). They are non-negotiable beliefs, linked to strong feelings, and can be seen within symbols, myths and heroes. Exploring who you see as a hero/heroine within each of the cultures that you inhabit can therefore be an easier way for you to identify what your cultural values are (Jandt, 2007). Figure 1.9 shows the cultural groups that you will be exploring. Box 1.8 shows how Sarah has applied her knowledge of her heroes and heroines to help articulate what her values are. If you look carefully you will note that not all of these values are compatible: her family and musical heroes break the rules, but her professional heroine is her mentor who strictly abides by policies. Being aware of these types of contradictions and tensions is an important first step in becoming a better communicator as you can weigh up what cultural influences may be impacting upon your interactions, and identify some alternative strategies that you may already have at your fingertips.

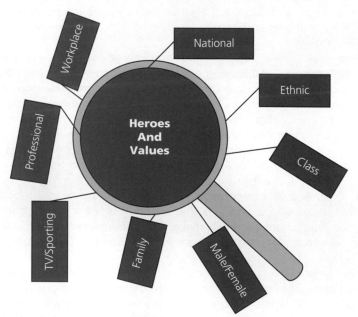

Figure 1.9: Cultural groups to which you belong

Culture	Your Identity	Hero/Heroine	What Values they Represent
National	British	Winston Churchill	Loyalty Never give in
Ethnic	Scottish	Robert the Bruce	Determination
Class	Working class	Union leaders	Never taking charity Hard work
Family	Daughter Sister Mother Niece Aunty	Uncle Fred (the rebel who left home to travel the world)	Ignoring the rules Adventurous Living life to the full
Hobby/TV/Sport	Music fan	Amy Winehouse	Musical talent Ignoring the rules
Profession	Nurse	Mary Seacole	Caring Dedication
Workplace	Accident and Emergency Nurse	Mentor	Knowledgeable Generous with time Caring Adhering to policy

Box 1.8: Sarah's cultural heroes and values

In music, a mixing desk is used to help to blend different aspects of a musical piece. Each element of the music is hidden within the piece as a whole, but the mixing desk can isolate each element to help unpick the complex melodies. The analogy will be used in the following sections to help you to understand how the different cultural dimensions shape the roles that you inhabit in your different cultural groups. You will also be asked to put into practice the knowledge about cultural dimensions by creating your own 'cultural dimension mixing desk'. You will be asked to think about the key cultural dimensions that were outlined in Figure 1.1 and apply them to yourself. To help you to do this you will be shown David's cultural mixing desk. At the end of all of the sections, you will be invited to record a summary of your own values just as

Sarah did in Box 1.8. As the concept of individualism and collectivism can be harder to identify within smaller groupings it has been omitted from the mixing desk. The factors that you will therefore be looking at within each of your groups are:

1. The degree to which the *cultural context* affects communication; in a high context culture, few words are needed to understand what is going on because you share background information, and in a low context culture, you need many words
2. The *power distance* between yourself and those in power. A high power distance means you feel you have little say in the decision-making process, a low power distance, you share the power
3. How much you try to *avoid uncertainty* or new situations – if you dislike uncertainty, you are high uncertainty avoidance
4. How much *activity* is expected from you when you're in that cultural setting – in a high activity level being busy is important; in low level, reflection and contemplation are important
5. How important it is to be aware of *time* – a high level means you are constantly clock watching, low level, time isn't so important
6. *Masculinity/Femininity* tendencies in communication

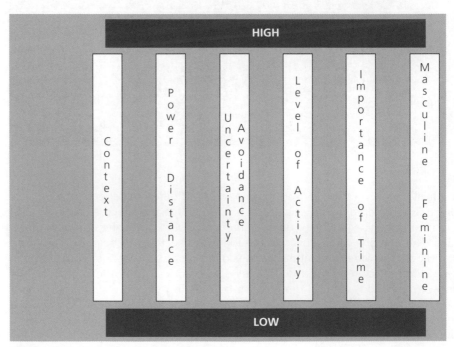

Figure 1.10: An example of a cultural mixing desk

The sections below apply these cultural dimensions to different cultural groupings:

1. Global culture (nationality)
2. Ethnicity
3. Class
4. Family
5. Social groups (for example hobby groups or religious groups)
6. Professional and organisational

GLOBAL/NATIONAL IDENTITY LENS

As noted previously, global cultures tend to be considered along an East/West orientation based upon historical patterns of thinking. As a quick reminder, Eastern cultures tend towards *high context* communication: people in a face to face setting know the status of the person that they are interacting with and adopt pre-set communication styles that show an appropriate level of respect. Children learn how to do this from an early age. Power is often concentrated in the hands of a few individuals who are relatively inaccessible to the rest of the population – they are therefore *high power distance* cultures. Since respect within communication is dependent upon knowing the status of the person with whom someone is interacting, care is taken to try to understand relative status positions to maintain harmony. There is therefore *high uncertainty avoidance* as not to know information may cause offence and loss of face. Orientation to *time* within the culture is generally *long term,* with decisions made in relation to not only current generations of the population but also to past and future generations. *Activity orientation* tends towards reflection – a *low* level of visible busyness. Examples of nations with this type of profile include Japan and China. An example of a cultural hero is Confucius with his teachings that promote order, faithfulness and selflessness (Jandt, 2007).

If you are from a Western culture, it is likely to be *individualistic* in nature. The needs of the individual and close family are more important than wider society. Communication orientation is *low context* in that members of the culture rely heavily upon words to deliver the message, which should be clear and explicit. Power is shared within democratic systems and therefore tends towards a *low power distance.* There is a *short term* orientation to time, with the past playing little role in decision making. Being busy and productive is important – there is *high activity orientation* and decisions are expected to be made quickly. There is a tendency towards *low uncertainty avoidance* and more comfort with risk taking. Examples of nations with this type of profile include the UK and USA (Hofstede, 1994; Hofstede, 1997; Jandt, 2007). An example of a hero within the USA that reflects the individualistic and low power distance values of the culture is John Wayne; the quintessential lone cowboy taking the law into his own hands.

David is from the UK, and his cultural mixing desk at the level of global/national culture reflects this Western influence as shown below:

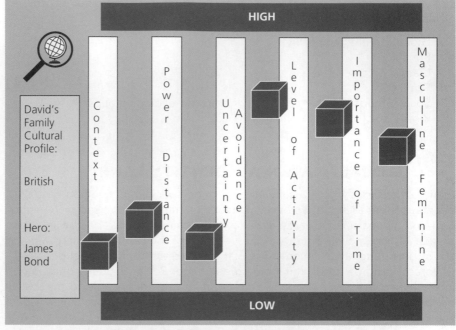

Figure 1.11: David's national cultural mixing desk profile

ETHNICITY LENS

Ethnicity and race are terms that are often used interchangeably and whose meanings shift over time. Ethnicity has at times been linked to biological origins, colour, country of origin, religious background or various combinations thereof (Jandt, 2007). Given these diverse influences, people within the same ethnic grouping may have multiple identities and ways of enacting their culture (Bailey, 2005). For the purposes of this book, it will be noted that we all have an ethnic background, but we may conceptualise it differently. The definition for ethnicity that we will ask you to use for your mixing desk is the one that you would usually choose if you were filling in a form that asked you for this information. When David fills in forms he ticks the boxes that indicate he is a white English person. This profile has many similarities with that of the majority of the national population; it therefore has many hidden norms and David is relatively blind to his own ethnicity. However, in his role as a social worker he is very culturally aware of the need to be sensitive to the needs of the different ethnic groups with whom he works. Staff who work in health and social care settings have to have knowledge of these type of cultural needs if they are to work effectively with people from different ethnic backgrounds (Laird, 2008; Raghavan, 2009; Kidd, 2010; Comas-Diaz, 2012). From an intercultural perspective, ethnicity becomes an issue primarily when the patterns of values and communication differ between participants within an interaction, regardless of which aspect of ethnicity causes the difference. Thus two white Americans who come from New York may struggle with communication if one communicates according to the norms of Jewish culture (fast, overlapping speech) and one according to the norms of the dominant, non-Jewish population (turn taking and waiting for the other person to finish speaking) (Tannen, 2005). However, both may tick the same ethnicity box (white American) if asked to do so within a formal survey. David's ethnic mixing desk profile is the same as his national profile.

CLASS LENS

Some national cultures include a class structure that clearly defines how an individual and their family are expected to relate to others. The class that a person is born into may affect the types of job that they are expected/allowed to engage in, how they are educated and how they are expected to communicate with others across classes. Examples of countries in which class structures are recognised to exist include India and Britain. The USA too can be viewed as having a class system based upon income and the type of work that members engage in (for example, blue collar/white collar (Philpsen, 1975)). The existence of class gives rise to sub cultures in which value systems and language are shared between members. For example, David has grown up in a working class family in which hard work (high activity levels), plain speaking and standing up for your rights and those of others in the same community are valued. There is shared knowledge and many in-jokes in the local community (high context communication). Within his family, there is a lot of value placed on the local community centre where many of the community projects are based. With high local unemployment levels, many people in the community do not experience pressures on time (low time importance). David feels he has some say in what happens at a local level (low power distance), even if he feels that his community is ignored by national government. At the community centre and within local groups, the language used includes swear words, and the type of communication style that is valued is masculine in nature. He was teased when his friends found out he wanted to be a social worker. There are very few people in his street who have attended university, and people are distrustful of those who have attended, generally preferring things to stay as they are (high uncertainty avoidance). The local heroes are stars of the football pitch who have practical, rather than

Think about your own ethnicity:

? **How do you describe yourself when you tick the ethnicity box on forms?**

? **Do you feel that your ethnicity reflects that of the majority of the population in the country in which you live?**

? **If not, using the cultural mixing desk to help you, identify how it may differ.**

? **How aware of your ethnicity are you when in your home country?**

? **How aware are you of your ethnicity if you mix with others from different ethnic backgrounds?**

Box 1.9: Reflections on your ethnicity

contemplative, intellectual skills. When he goes to work and attends meetings, he is very conscious that the kind of language that is appropriate at the community centre would be inappropriate in that setting. He is conscious that many of his service users who come from a similar background feel very out of place in meetings, with their formal structures, academic language and time constraints. His class cultural mixing desk differs from his national culture mixing desk:

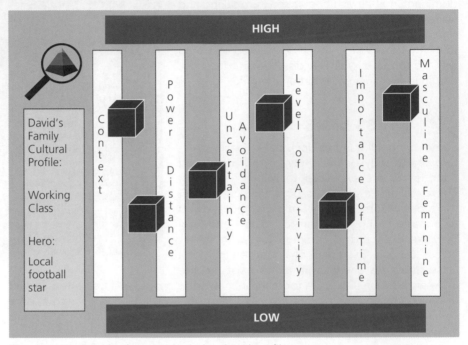

Figure 1.12: David's class mixing desk cultural profile

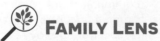 **FAMILY LENS**

The ways that families are structured are affected by the wider cultural contexts within which they develop: nation, ethnicity and class. These cultural values affect the ways in which masculine and feminine roles are viewed, how parents and children interact, and how these traditions are passed down through the generations. Individual personality traits also become more influential as the cultural group in question becomes smaller (Jandt, 2007; Neuliep, 2009). David lives with his mother, father and younger sister in the family home. They are a close knit family that share many values such as loyalty to one another, supporting each other during crises and putting others in the family first when joint decisions need to be made. The family share a lot of knowledge and values that they would be hard pressed to put into words and can be considered as a high context culture with low power distance tendencies. The family believe that it's important to relax together at home and over meals; busyness in the house is generally avoided (low level of activity), but woe betide anyone who is late for the family meal (high importance of time)! The family are caring (high femininity trait). Generally, the family hate things to change (high uncertainty avoidance). The family heroine is Aunty Sue who took in her sister's children when she was ill to avoid them having to go into care. David's family cultural mixing desk is illustrated below:

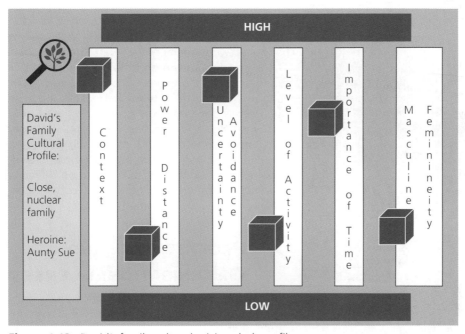

Figure 1.13: David's family cultural mixing desk profile

 ## Social Groupings Lens

Social groups may be formal groups (such as the guiding movement or church groups), or informal groups such as street gangs and friendship groups. These types of groups may develop highly specialised language systems **(argot)** that help to define group membership. Knowledge of what language to use, and how and when to use it can help to define those who are inside and outside the culture (Jandt, 2007; Labov, 1972). David is a member of many different cultural groups, all of which have specific value systems to which he is expected to conform, and which use different specialised words. Whilst there are some similarities in the value bases that he adheres to there are also differences. He is

Culture	Your Identity	Your Hero	What Values they Represent
National			
Ethnic			
Class			
Family			
Hobby/TV/ Sports			
Profession			
Workplace			

Have a go at filling in the table.

? Think about how you would describe your identity in relation to each of the cultural groups.

? Which heroes/heroines can you identify?

? What values do you think they may represent?

? Which cultural heroes/heroines are easy to identify and which are hard?

? Are all of the cultural values in your table compatible?

Box 1.10: Your cultural values and heroes/heroines

Fill in the cultural mixing desk shown below.

? Use a dark coloured pen to mark your cultural dimensions for an encounter with one of your friends.

? Use a red pen to mark the dimensions affecting your professional role as you interact with a service user at work.

a member of the local Church of England, which has stylised formats for its services (high uncertainty avoidance), follows traditional Christian values and emphasises the importance of reflection and prayer (stillness is valued). The cultural hero is Jesus. He used to be a member of the scouts, which were activity oriented. His scouting cultural hero used to be Baden-Powell and now his hero is the Chief Scout and TV personality Bear Grylls. In terms of the communication styles of both of those groups, swearing is taboo. He still helps out at scouts occasionally if they are short of adult volunteers, but prefers to go to the local pub to hang out with his mates to watch the football. There he joins in the arguments about football teams, swears along with his mates and looks suitably tough if he is teased about his job. The pub hero is Joe, who can down 12 pints of beer and who once knocked two teeth out of a biker who came to the pub and insulted his girlfriend. The culture mixing desk for each of those groupings looks very different, but he has no difficulty in switching between cultures and communication styles.

PROFESSIONAL AND ORGANISATIONAL LENSES

Professional groups and organisations have mission statements, policies and other documentation that outline the espoused values of the culture. They use specialised communication systems to share those values with others inside and outside of the system (Schein, 2010). These are the overt cultural norms. The remaining chapters in this book are designed to help you to think about the hidden dimensions of communication within those cultures that may be preventing the espoused aims from being applied to people who are communicatively vulnerable. David's cultural mixing desk will not be shown in this section as it may influence your own reflections. Instead, to help you to start thinking about these issues you are asked to fill in Box 1.10, which outlines the varied and possibly conflicting cultural values that you hold, just as Sarah did. You are also asked to compare and contrast how you think your communication with friends and service users differs by using the mixing desk in Figure 1.14. It is likely that you will have many different examples to select from, so choose one that reflects an 'average' encounter.

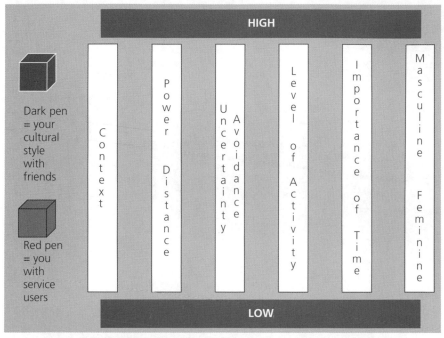

Figure 1.14: Your cultural mixing desk: friends and service users

CULTURE IS COMMUNICATION

Our cultural dimensions and values influence every aspect of our communication, usually without us being consciously aware of it (Scollon *et al.*, 2012; Ziviani *et al.*, 2004). The pictures below illustrate this point by taking a very simple interaction: that of asking for a drink. They are linked to a video created by Communicate2U that shows how varied communication can be in different cultural settings. Have a look at the video first, then look at the photos in the box that show people interacting in different situations and think about how you would ask for a drink in the same settings. This example has been selected, because as you will find out in later chapters, this activity can be of primary importance to service users and carers. Poor communication in something this simple can be indicative of much deeper rooted cultural communication inequities. Communicate2U members have often found that health and social care staff are very poor at meeting their basic needs. Two members of the group had their health put at severe risk because of staff communication failures in this domain. It is important to them that you view the video to learn from their experiences. If you only rely on reading these academic words, you are likely to be part of the problem, rather than the solution, so please ensure that you take a few moments to undertake the activity they have prepared for you.

Watch the video that shows you people asking for a drink in different cultural settings. As you watch, think about the following:

?   **What cultural norms are being enacted?**

?   **What values are people showing by acting that way?**

?   **What role does context play in the communication? (For example, how much background knowledge does the other person have?)**

?   **How much of the communication requires explicit use of words and how much is implicit or through body language?**

Now look at the pictures below that show people asking for a drink in different cultural settings and ask yourself the same questions as you think how you personally would get a drink in these settings.

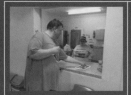
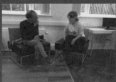
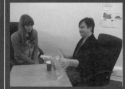
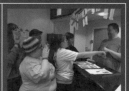

| In a foreign country where you don't speak the language | At home, asking a close family member to get you your usual drink | At work in a formal meeting | Out with friends |

How do your strategies compare with those shown in the video?

Box 1.11: Culture and communication: asking for a drink in different cultural settings

As the activity in Box 1.11 illustrates, we can do the same activity in many different ways depending on the role that we inhabit and the culture in which we enact it. As we do so, we alter our communication styles in ways that reflect our values and attitudes. As social beings we are capable of holding multiple attitudes at any one time, many of which may actually be in conflict (Berger *et al.*, 1969). Therefore, an important element of communication from a cultural perspective is knowing which value system to act on within a given setting. If you doubt the importance of this, try speaking to your parents or tutor in the same way that you speak to your friends and see how long it takes for them to correct you! Problems with clashing cultural patterns can result in major communication difficulties such as culture shock and culture clashes.

BARRIERS TO EFFECTIVE INTERCULTURAL COMMUNICATION

Culture shock is a term that is used to explain the difficulties that people experience when they are unprepared to function in a new culture that is very different to their own. It is the type of experience that you may have had when on holiday in a foreign country where everything appears confusing. Some people enjoy this type of challenge, whilst others may find it stressful. Culture shock is generally associated with the global level of culture (Jandt, 2007; Neuliep, 2009; Scollon et al., 2012). When we travel to a different country or meet others from a different national or ethnic background, at some level we often expect there to be some differences, even if these still come as a shock. When we meet people who look very much like ourselves, however, our cultural differences are generally hidden. These problems can also occur when people from smaller, **non-dominant cultural groups** interact with people from the dominant cultural group: here it is referred to as a **culture clash**. The resultant feelings of anxiety, stress or anger are often blamed on the other person being unreasonable, rather than recognising that there is a difference in cultural expectations (Hall, 1959). In hospital or social care settings, staff are members of the **dominant culture**, and service users and carers are members of the non-dominant culture. When Sarah and Jeff met briefly in the hospital, their encounter could be viewed in terms of a culture clash. The feelings experienced by the less culturally dominant person tend to be strong and negative; they may therefore have an influence far beyond the brief moments of the face to face encounter. Avoiding such clashes is an important step in reducing the risk that vulnerable clients face when interacting with health and social care staff.

The ability to communicate effectively across cultures of any level is termed **intercultural competence** (Neuliep, 2009). A competent intercultural communicator is able to recognise the multiple cultural identities that people may inhabit. They use this knowledge to negotiate cultural meanings so that both their own communication goals and those of the people with whom they interact are respected. The skill sets that are required in order to achieve competence include intercultural sensitivity, self-awareness, flexibility and social skills (Chen et al., 1996b), tolerance and openness to new experiences (Jandt, 2007). The barriers to intercultural competence include:

- Anxiety
- Assuming similarity where there is difference
- Ethnocentrism (judging other people's culture negatively according to one's own values)
- Stereotyping and prejudice
- Non-verbal misinterpretations
- Language as a barrier (Barna, 1997)

If you have taken part in the exercises in this chapter, you should now be in a position to recognise the different cultures to which you belong, some of the values that you hold in relation to those cultures, and how your communication styles may vary as you enact your cultural roles. You should also now be aware that you have a wealth of different values and communication styles that you enact in different settings. This is the foundation for the chapters that follow, which will help to address the barriers outlined above. If you haven't undertaken the exercises, it may be worth reflecting on why you felt it unnecessary, or not of primary importance to do so.

CHAPTER SUMMARY

Every time you interact with another person, you do so in relation to patterns of communication that you have learned from the many different cultural groups of which you are a member. The vast majority of those patterns will be invisible to you, and that lack of knowledge means that whilst you and others like you may judge your communication to be good, some of the most vulnerable people in health and social care settings may find it to be poor. People can be vulnerable for many reasons – for example, because they have a learning disability, mental health problem or don't have the same first language. Learning more about the patterns of communication that you use in the many cultural groups to which you belong is the first step to reducing the risk of culture clashes with people who are communicatively vulnerable. Subsequent chapters will argue that many staff in health and social care are prone to ethnocentrism, non-verbal misinterpretation, stereotyping and prejudice when interacting with their most vulnerable clients. They perform these acts whilst fully believing that they are complying with the positive stated values of their profession and organisation, and they do so because they are unable to see the cultural world view of others, and cannot articulate their own conflicting cultural perspectives and values. Viewing communication from an intercultural perspective could help to reduce the risk that this type of cultural view poses.

EASY READ CHAPTER SUMMARY

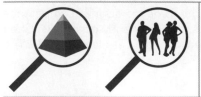	We all belong to many different groups. We can think about these groups as cultures.
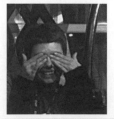	In different cultural groups, we communicate differently. We may not see this.

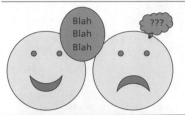	If people from different cultural groups meet, communication may be hard.
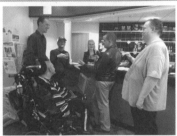	Learning about our own cultures can help to improve our communication skills. This helps when we meet people who communicate in ways that are different to ours. This is called **intercultural competence**.
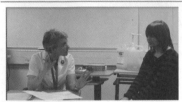 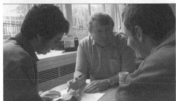	Staff in health or social care jobs need these skills to communicate well with people who find using words hard. This book will help people to get better at **intercultural competence**.

VALUES, POWER AND COMMUNICATION

Aims

By the end of this chapter you will be able to:

➡ Identify what types of power you have in different cultural settings

➡ Compare and contrast your power with that of service users

➡ Describe how power differentials may cause people to be vulnerable within communication exchanges

➡ Use a model to map how the identification of power issues may improve interaction with people who may be communicatively vulnerable

INTRODUCTION

Trying to pin power down to one definition actually highlights one of the key points of this book – words are slippery things that can't always easily communicate meaning. Theorists and practitioners alike will use terms such as 'power' in many different ways, using different language and concepts to frame their ideas (Croom, 2012; Haugaard, 2002; Wittgenstein, 1967). These differences in views can make it difficult to understand the concept when reading about the topic from a theoretical standpoint. The theory can make power seem an abstract concept that has limited place in the real world. However, most of us at some point in our lives have known what it feels like to be powerful (feels wonderful) or disempowered with little control over what happens to us (feels horrible). We understand power from a practical and emotional perspective, even if we may struggle to explain why we feel the way that we do about the situation. This may be how service users feel at times. As you will discover as you read through this chapter, power is often inextricably linked to knowledge. If you wish to empower the service users that you work with, you need to know what types of power you actually hold, and how that power is shared (or not as the case may be). In Chapter 1 you learned that failing to see hidden dimensions of culture can cause professionals to inadvertently place vulnerable service users at risk. The ways in which power is distributed was highlighted as a key cultural dimension. This chapter explores that dimension in more depth and gives you practical techniques to map how your knowledge and power may impact upon communication with vulnerable service users.

Aspects of Power

In keeping with the focus on culture that is central to this book, power is argued to be intrinsically linked to cultural values and ideologies (Hofstede, 1997; Lukes, 1974). In Chapter 1, you were introduced to the concept of high and low power distance cultures. When there is a high power distance, power is held centrally by a few people, and where there is a low power distance, a greater number of people share in the decision-making processes. You were invited to undertake exercises to help you to understand about your own cultural values and patterns. The exercises were:

- **Box 1.10 – Cultural Values and Heroes**
- **Figure 1.14 – Your Cultural Mixing Desk**

You may find it helpful to review these exercises before reading the next sections as they will help you to link the theoretical concepts to practical examples.

Thus far we have talked about how power is shared within cultures, but we haven't yet said what it is actually made up of. This is particularly important to unravel if we consider power in the context of health and social care. Empowerment is often cited as a professional value in the UK and other Western cultures (NMC, COT, 2015; 2008; Sasso *et al.*, 2008), and this implies some sort of power sharing. However, it is difficult to share something if you can't identify what you have that the other person lacks. Box 2.1 gives you some examples of types of power that have been identified by some key theorists in the left and how they are used by professionals David and Sarah who you met in Chapter 1 (Box 1.2). You will also see how this has the potential to impact upon their service users.

The examples shown in Box 2.1 also illustrate two further key concepts associated with power: the degree of freedom that individuals have to act within the structures that already exist (agency and structure), and the degree to which they are prepared to share the power that they know they hold (zero sum and generative views of power).

The amount of freedom that people have to act varies and to help you to identify what may empower or constrain you as a professional, this is explained here in terms of **agency** and **structure**. **Agency** may be considered as the

Aspect of power	Power and theorists	Links to professionals (Sarah and David)	Links to service users
1. Using resources and strategies	People in power can use resources and strategies to achieve their goals (Machiavelli). They can use power to manipulate the less powerful without them realising this (Marx) and they have the capacity to achieve outcomes (Giddens, Parsons).	Sarah saw that the waiting area in her department was drab, boring and added to the stress of patients. Managers did not listen to her requests to address this. However, she knew that patient complaints were monitored by managers and used this knowledge to achieve her goal. She encouraged patients who commented on the décor to fill in a form. The area was upgraded.	When Jeff attended the hospital, he found a bright and cheerful place to wait in. He enjoyed looking at the pictures in the magazines whilst he waited his turn. This reduced his levels of stress.
2. The power of language	The ability to articulate ideas and debate them effectively is a form of power (Habermas). Those who are more effective in their use of language have power over those who are less articulate (Bourdieu).	As a social worker, David often has to support families and service users to understand the complex rules and paperwork that affect their rights to support. In meetings with other professionals he tries to support them to speak for themselves, but may speak up on their behalf if they seem to be struggling to follow the discussion.	Many service users and families get worried by the formal letters they are sent. They feel out of place in the meetings where professionals use complex words. They rely on David to translate letters for them and are grateful when he advocates on their behalf. However, as the system does not change, this means that they remain dependent upon him and professionals like him.
3. The power of being a professional	Professionals have the power to create and shape the role that service users play (Foucault).	Sarah's workplace generally expects service users to conform to the role of a patient who is seeking help from knowledgeable experts in an emergency. David's work place views service users as experts in their own experiences.	Jeff finds it very confusing. Sometimes he is expected to give his own ideas, and sometimes he is expected to keep quiet and just listen. This can even happen in the same room if he talks to different people. If he does the wrong thing, others may get cross – this stresses him out.

(Bachrach *et al.*, 1963; Bachrach *et al.*, 1970; Bachrach *et al.*, 1962; Bourdieu, 1991; Clegg, 1989; Dahl, 1968; Foucault, 1965; Foucault, 1985; Giddens, 1984; Haugaard, 2002; Jackson, 2004; Lukes, 1974; Wrong, 1979)

Box 2.1: Aspects of power impacting upon professionals and service users

motivations that drive individuals to act in the way that they do, and the degree of freedom that they have to act upon those drives. In example 1, Sarah was highly motivated to try to make the experience of being in hospital less stressful for the service users. However, the existing organisational **structure** contained forces (such as managers) that prevented her from having free choice in her actions. Knowing how the structure worked enabled her to be quite Machiavellian in her planning. The service users in theory had the power to make the change to the environment, but in practice lacked this knowledge and so didn't use it effectively. Sarah was quite effective in manipulating this situation for their benefit. Knowledge is powerful. Agency and structure don't only work at the level of organisational or professional culture; they also work at the national level of culture. Both Sarah and David are greatly affected by the government that constructs the health and welfare systems within which they work, and that determines how they should persuade people to adhere to policies or adopt reforms (Taylor Gooby, 2008a; Taylor Gooby, 2008b). At the national cultural level, some cultures (such as the USA) may implicitly expect a higher level of individual responsibility and choice (agency) to be adopted by people in relation to their own well-being. Other cultures may have structural precepts that encourage a more group approach to taking responsibility for those who are unwell or in need (for example, some Eastern cultures). Some cultures (such as the UK) adopt a mixed system, whereby there is an increasing emphasis on people making their own choices and taking responsibility for actions (agency) within a state welfare system (structure) that may in reality limit the choices that are available. Example three shows how both systems may exist side by side, and how confusing this can be for service users who are then not sure how they are supposed to act.

Another key theoretical element that will affect us on a very personal level is how much power we think actually exists, and whether we consider it to be finite. If we think of power as being something that will diminish if we give some of it away, we are adopting a **zero sum** view of power. People who

Thinking about Agency and Structure

Think about a large library in which you have studied.

Agency = You have the power to move around and do things within some parts of the building. You may be motivated to do so because you wish to learn, or you want to pass exams to earn money.

Structure = Your power to move around will be limited by factors outside of your control. Examples include the physical structure (you can't walk through walls!), or limitations that management may have put on you (you are not allowed to access all areas).

Now think about an organisation in which you have worked or been on placement.

? **What things do you have control over?**

? **What factors limit your power to act?**

How comfortable are you about sharing power?

ZERO SUM VIEW

? **Is power like a cake? If you give away a slice, there's less for you?**

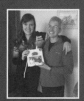

GENERATIVE VIEW

? **Is power like love? Giving it away to others creates more?**

Box 2.2: Your experiences of agency, structure and power sharing hold this view of power may be unwilling to share the power that they do have, for fear of losing it. An alternative view of power is that of it being **generative** – sharing power generates more power (Haugaard, 2002). People who hold this view may be more comfortable with power sharing. Both Sarah and David are comfortable with power sharing to some degree and tend towards a generative view of power. However, they both work within organisations in which the ultimate power is usually held by professionals and managers who hold a more zero sum view of power sharing. Example 2 in Box 2.1 illustrates one of the ways in which this occurs: professionals control the language that dominates the organisation, and they can determine how much and what type of information gets filtered out to service users. Neither Sarah nor David are fully conscious of the degree to which this occurs. By advocating for service users they feel they are empowering individuals. They overlook the fact that this prevents larger structural and organisational changes from taking place that may make it easier for service users to get the information in an accessible format. These types of changes could ultimately facilitate self advocacy. Self advocacy would empower service users, but may also mean that they have information that could be used to challenge existing structures, which managers who hold a zero sum view of power would find threatening. Power that is hidden is insidious and can therefore deceive even those who wield it. Making power visible can help professionals to be conscious of how much power they are holding and how much they are choosing to share with others. To help you see this, we are going to use the three dimensions of power identified by Lukes (1974). This gives you a practical way of outlining what type of power you as professional may hold, what may constrain your uses of that power, and how you deal with power differentials within face to face interactions (Avery, 2007).

The First Dimension of Power – Power Over Others (Agency)

The first dimension of power is the ability to make someone do something that they otherwise would not have done (Dahl, 1968). Sarah exercised this type of power when she asked service users to fill in complaint forms. David exercised this type of power when he supported people to speak up at a meeting when they found it difficult. You will use this type of power on a daily basis – whether it's getting someone to get you a drink, or to help you with a task. In all of these examples, the end result is quite positive for the people exercising the power. Jeff, the service user with a learning disability, also had power over others in the hospital setting when he went off wandering to try to find a friendly nurse: he made them escort him back to the bay. In this case, however, he made people come out of their usual work role, which annoyed them and caused them to be cross with him; the experience was not pleasant for either party. For this type of power to be exercised positively therefore, people have to have strategies in place.

Think about the strategies that you use to try to get someone to make you a drink:

- How do you know to try to use them?
- How skilled are you at using them?
- How effective are they?

You are more likely to be able to achieve your goal if you know a bit about what motivates the other person (agency) or the social structures that surround the activity. For example you may use guilt (I made you a drink last time), or the social convention of turn taking (I'll make the next one) to exercise your power. You have resources at your disposal which you can utilise to make the other person react. Jeff had fewer resources at his disposal when he was making his request for support in an unfamiliar setting, and was far less effective in gaining a positive outcome.

Differences in the amounts of power that individuals hold are, at the most basic level, explained by differences in the amount and type of resources that they hold. These may include the following domains:

- Societal or cultural respect for the role occupied
- Well-being
- Skills
- Knowledge of the culture and environment in which the encounter takes place
- Affection
- Control over financial resources
- Knowledge as to how systems operate
- Control over jobs
- Control over sources of information

Family Cultural Lens

Think of your own family unit. Pick someone in the family who you feel is in a position of power. Think of a time when that power has been used with you and you have not been happy. Consider the resource list opposite and reflect:

? **Does that person have more power than you in all of the resources listed?**

? **Is that difference large or small?**

? **Are there other resources that you feel they have used that are not listed?**

? **How effective are they in using their resources in achieving their aims?**

? **How do you feel when this occurs?**

Box 2.3: Power and disempowerment in your family setting

However, access to resources is not the only factor that influences how much power an individual has. The scope of power (over how many people that power can be exerted) and the intensity of the effect are also important aspects (Dahl, 1968; Wrong, 1979). In reality, individuals may have theoretical access to power, but lack the capability to exercise it effectively. Since being in a position of power is comfortable, we may not notice the power that we exert. However, as the introduction to this chapter noted, we soon notice when we are disempowered. Have a go at the exercise in Box 2.3, which explores power under the family cultural lens and asks you to reflect upon a time when you were disempowered. This will prepare you for thinking about power and resources that affect service users in health and social care settings.

 Professional/Organisational Lens and Agency

Organisations utilise many different mechanisms to organise and control how much agency (the first dimension of power) its members have. The hierarchical structure, communication lines and degrees to which individuals are enabled to

control the decisions that occur within their working lives are the mechanisms that determine power distribution (Schein, 2010). The degree to which professionals in health and social care take an interest in, and are aware of, these power distributions varies (Apter, 2014; Gilbert *et al.*, 2003; McCarthy *et al.*, 2008; Phillips, 2005; Rogers, 2012; Wilkinson *et al.*, 1999). You may already have been taught to frame your knowledge of power within a specific theoretical framework, or you may not have fully considered power before. In either case, we will ask you now to consider the organisation within which you work (or the type of organisations within which you may have future placements or employment), and your profession purely in terms of the resources outlined above. Depending upon the situation and your relative position within the setting, there may be times when you feel you have a relatively large degree of power (for example, when your skills are those that are in demand), and other times when you feel relatively powerless (for example, at a meeting dominated by professionals who have very different knowledge bases to your own). Now use the mixing desk in Figure 2.1 to consider how your power base in relation to some of the resources listed above relates to that of the average person who is likely to access your service or profession seeking support. The level of skill refers to the skill needed to undertake the task for which the person has been referred to your service, cultural knowledge relates to how much the person knows about how the organisation and the professional functions, and the control of finances or information relates to how much influence the person has in deciding where and in what format the organisational resources are distributed.

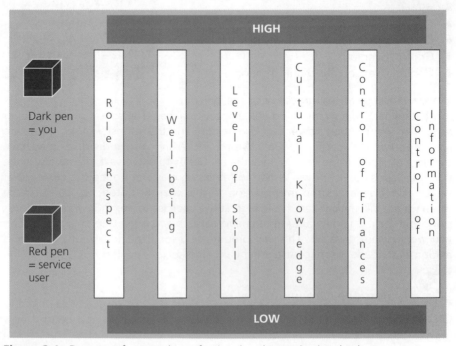

Figure 2.1: Degrees of agency in professional and organisational cultures

You may work within cultures and organisations that support an empowerment agenda, and encourage service users to be experts in managing their own conditions (Laverack, 2005; Scheckel *et al.*, 2009). You may also work with people who are not only service users coming to you for support, but who are also professionals in health and social care in their day jobs. However, in relation to the vast majority of service users who enter those organisations, and even those with additional knowledge, you will occupy a relative position of power. You have access to the following resources:

- Knowledge of organisational policies, procedures and priorities
- Knowledge as to the range of services that you are able to offer (and which you cannot)
- Knowing who to go to for more information
- Knowing who is effective at getting things done in the organisation
- Technical language used by other professionals
- Knowing how to find your way around buildings and access services (such as drinks facilities)

All of this knowledge will have been communicated to you in one form or another – whether in books, leaflets or through the spoken word. You may use similar mechanisms to pass some of this knowledge on to your service users. If you struggle to access this knowledge yourself because of a specific learning difficulty, sensory impairment or lack of knowledge of the first language, you too may feel disempowered when interacting with other professionals within an organisation. As example two at the start of this chapter (Box 2.1) illustrated, knowing the language and controlling what form it takes is a hidden and very powerful tool. If you were to redo the mixing desk exercise (Figure 2.1) for a service user such as Jeff who has very limited access to word-based resources, you would find that the power differential becomes vastly increased, regardless of where you place yourself in the power hierarchy.

> *They make me go to meetings then they talk about me like I'm not there.*
>
> *If I go to the doctor or the nurse, they try and make me sit on the chair. I don't like sitting on a chair unless there's a table in front of me because I have a phobia.*
>
> *I have to get up at the same time every day even if I don't want to. Some days I don't have to go out early so I want to stay in bed but I can't.*

Communicate2U quotation 2.1: Service users' experiences of disempowerment

Members of Communicate2U have had many negative experiences of disempowerment of this nature in both health and social care settings. As the quotations shown above illustrate, professionals will often make them do things that they otherwise would not have done. They may be expected to attend meetings in which the language used is inaccessible and they are ignored for the major-ity of the time. They will be expected to sit in places allocated by professionals, or to stick to timetables that are convenient for the professionals running the organisation, not the service users that are living there. The examples above are a small fraction of the daily experiences of disempowerment that are faced by people whose access to power resources is limited. Few of the professionals concerned will have intended to have this effect, and most will probably never realise that they did. They took their power for granted, and did not recognise how many resources they actually controlled.

Ultimately, whether consciously or unconsciously, you control the decision as to whether you share the knowledge of resources that may be hidden to the service user, how much to share, or whether you keep that knowledge to your-self. Earlier in this chapter you were asked to consider how comfortable you were with sharing power. Take a moment now to look again at the mixing desk that you completed in Figure 2.1 that outlined your power compared to that of ser-vice users. How much of the power that you have outlined do you really share in practice, and is that a conscious decision or an unconscious one? The exercises in this section have been designed to try to bring the unconscious decisions relating to power to your conscious awareness. Once you have awareness of what power you possess, you then have to decide how to distribute it. The next section explores some of the mechanisms by which the more powerful individual can intentionally and consciously retain power.

The Second Dimension of Power – Bias

A more powerful person can dominate another not only by making them do things, but also by limiting the choices that are available to them (Bachrach et al., 1962). They can decide what items get put onto the agenda for discussion, and which items are omitted. The person in power can therefore ensure that items that have the potential to be disadvantageous to him or her can either fail to make the agenda in the first place, or can be postponed indefinitely. Non-decision making is therefore a subtle and deliberate exercising of power (Bachrach et al., 1963). In Box 2.1, Sarah experienced this type of power when her requests to manage-ment for environmental upgrades were ignored: minor funding requests from staff had low priority and could be postponed. She overcame this by using her knowledge of the agenda as she knew that service user complaints always had to be addressed. Service users, however, had no knowledge that this agenda even existed. In Sarah's case, knowledge of the agenda gave her power. Organisations and professions have many different (and possibly conflicting) agendas running simultaneously. There will be agendas that are made public, and some that are kept private. Service users therefore may only have very limited knowledge of all the issues that affect them. As Tony's case scenario in Box 2.4 illustrates, know-ing what can be put on the agenda and knowing how to deal with non-decision making can have a profound effect on the quality of service that people receive.

Committees, red tape, retaining control over what is deemed to be impor-tant or not are all very effective mechanisms by which power can be retained (Haugaard, 2002). These aspects of power are by their very nature often hidden

Tony has very limited movement. He communicates by using his eyes to show an assistant which word in a book he wishes to use, or he uses small movements to activate an electronic voice aid. It takes him quite a long time to access each word in the book or on the voice aid, but he is able to understand everything that goes on around him. For many years, Tony lived in a care home and was frustrated at the group nature of the lifestyle he experienced. Initially he was unaware of a funding scheme (individual budget) that could support a move to independent living. Tony had a complex care package at the home, and had regular meetings in which members of health and social care staff got together to discuss his needs. Although staff were aware of his frustrations, the option of an individual budget was not raised for some time. The package in place was working, and changing things would have required a lot of work. Once the individual budget was mentioned, Tony repeatedly expressed the wish to move into his own place. At subsequent meetings, this issue was sometimes put onto the agenda for discussion, but it was often omitted. If it was discussed, staff would often suggest that more information was needed, and would shelve any action until someone in the group had accessed it. On some occasions, the information was out of date by the time it had been brought back to the group, and the process was restarted. This went on for years. However, Tony would not let the item be dropped from the agenda. When a new staff member joined, they saw what was happening and supported Tony to get his voice heard. They insisted upon action points and dates to be added to the agenda and eventually Tony succeeded in his aim to get his own place.

Box 2.4: Case Scenario: Tony

from those on the receiving end – if you don't even know that it's an option, you aren't aware that you're missing out. In Tony's case, the issues regarding control were insidious. The culture was one in which meetings were designed to include service users (to tick the box for empowerment), but the real agenda was controlled by the staff. If controlling the agenda is a routine part of the culture, those who are nominally part of the power mechanisms may also fail to fully appreciate what is happening as it is a hidden cultural norm. The arrival of a new staff member exposed the norm and their persistence shifted the balance of power behind the agenda so that it worked for Tony, rather than the institution.

We have all experienced being on the receiving end of an agenda set by someone else, and we may or may not have been aware of this at the time. The exercise in Box 2.5 is designed to help you think about how you were affected by the second dimension of power at home when you were a child, and therefore likely to be in a disempowered position in the family. Work through the exercise and consider the impact of agendas on how much choice you actually had, and how you felt about this.

People who access health and social care services as service users are constantly affected by this second dimension of power. Professionals usually have a greater knowledge as to what options are available within a service and they determine which ones to offer and which ones not to mention. Sometimes, they set up power sharing mechanisms to bring managers, staff and service users together (for example, in partnership boards or patient liaison organisations) to discuss issues, but the creation of such mechanisms does not of itself ensure power distribution. This will depend upon the agendas that drive such meetings. When organisational cultures are framed around an overt agenda of power sharing, control of what goes onto the agenda can also be shared (Finlay *et al.*,

Family Cultural Lens

Think back to a time when you were a child and your family was deciding how to spend time at the weekend, and you felt you were not listened to (if you struggle with this, you may think of an alternative, for example, who decided what was put on the table to eat).

? **What kind of activities were put on the agenda?**

? **Who put them there?**

? **Were there any things that you tried to put on the agenda that were not taken seriously?**

? **If your ideas were listened to, how did that feel?**

? **If your ideas were ignored, how did that feel?**

Other cultural lenses:

? **Do the types of issues outlined above still occur in other areas of your life such as friendship groups or work?**

? **How does it feel?**

Box 2.5: Your experiences of agendas and power in the family

2008c; Stevens *et al.*, 2011). This offers the potential for concerns to be raised and addressed before the issues become too problematic. Organisational cultures in which control over the agenda is in reality retained by a few powerful individuals do not have this facility. In such situations the overt agenda may be one of empowerment, but the hidden agenda is one in which professionals seek to retain power. Inquiries into poor practice often uncover just how difficult it can be for service users or families to get an item onto the agenda if the organisation is unwilling to explore that topic (Mencap, 2013; Mencap, 2006). In the Mencap cases that sought to expose the poor treatment of people with a learning disability, carers had to use the power of national organisations in order to make the issue of poor care an item for discussion. Only when external publicity made it problematic for the health or social care organisation concerned did it become an agenda item within the organisation. By this time, numerous vulnerable individuals had been harmed by poor care. Failing to get the service user and carer issues onto the agenda at an early stage also caused harm to the organisations as they were then damaged by negative publicity. It could therefore be argued that sharing power over what goes on the organisational agenda could be an important factor in protecting both service users and organisations in the long term.

Implicit within all of the discussion above is an assumption that everybody can understand the form of communication that frames the agenda: that people can read material to understand what the issues are, that they can use words to articulate their ideas, and that there is a level playing field in terms of the language resources that each person can access. This is a fundamental assumption that must be challenged, for unless the agenda is available in a form that is accessible to all, professionals and organisations will always control the agenda – regardless of what may be written on it. If people lack this capacity, then those in charge of the written and spoken agenda may feel it prudent to make decisions on behalf of those who are not capable. It could be argued that organisations or professions may feel that they need to control the agenda in order to protect themselves or others. For example, they may feel that lay people do not understand the more complex issues or that others who are not present at meetings also need to be considered. This leads us to the third dimension of power – that of considering in whose interests a decision is made.

The Third Dimension of Power – Interests Served

The first two dimensions of power have concentrated on how individuals or groups control resources or decision making. This assumes a mainly conscious and intentional act on the part of those in power, but, as we have already seen, these acts can become part of the culture and therefore hard to see. Lukes (1974) argued that the hidden social structures that affect how people control one another should be made more explicit. He therefore added a third dimension to the two already outlined – consideration as to whose interests are served when resources are distributed and agendas are constructed. Central to this dimension is consideration as to whether there is conflict between parties. Conflict is either observable and obvious, or hidden (latent). A latent conflict is an issue in which the less powerful person or group is unaware that their interests are not being best served, and should they gain this knowledge, obvious conflict may result.

Very roughly speaking, Lukes framed his third dimension of power around the following points:

- Differing parties may have interests that conflict or do not conflict
- Differing parties may perceive there to be subjective interests and real interests
- Where there is no legitimate power and there is conflict, there may be coercion or force
- Where there is legitimate power and conflict, there may be manipulation
- Where there is legitimate authority and no conflict of interests, there may be persuasion/encouragement, but no issues of power

These points are summarised in Figure 2.2:

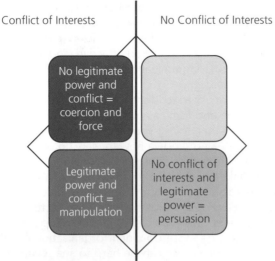

Figure 2.2: Summary of the impact of conflict of interests and legitimacy of authority on power (after Lukes, 1974)

Lukes argued that where there is no conflict of interest, no power is exercised. He also argued that there may be subjective interests and real interests that are perceived differently by different people. We'll put these issues to the side for the moment to focus upon issues of conflicting interests and power.

Those who are more powerful can potentially dominate the less powerful by making them believe in values and ideologies which are actually contrary to their best interests. They may make use of control of the agenda to further their own issues. In Tony's case scenario (Box 2.4), staff were presenting an ideology of safety linked to maintaining the status quo of life in an institution. This conflicted with Tony's beliefs about being allowed to take the risks associated with independent living that he felt would enhance his quality of life. It could be argued that the people who benefitted most from the status quo were the staff in the organisation who were funded to provide the place, and whose work was less onerous if things stayed as they were. As soon as Tony had information about funding that supported his imagined independent future, latent conflicts became observable conflicts within meetings. This illustrates the close links between social structures, the knowledge that people within those structures have, and power. In this case, staff with legitimate authority had the power to manipulate the less powerful person into doing things they would otherwise not have done.

People can make others do things without necessarily having legitimate authority to undertake these acts. In this case, they may use coercion or force. A scandal in the UK at Winterbourne View (a residential unit for people with a learning disability) illustrates these aspects of power. Many residents experienced emotional or physical abuse at the hands of staff, and their families had no power to remove their relative. The interests of the less powerful service users and family were therefore in conflict with those of the authorities when staff stepped outside of their legitimate boundaries to use coercion or force. The serious case review into the scandal noted one staff member commenting that the only language a patient understood was force (Flynn, 2012). Abuse and force became a part of the cultural norm. These practices were justified as appropriate interventions by professionals who lacked effective (and legitimate) communication and therapeutic skills. Communication is an important issue when consideration of best interests arises.

In Chapter 1 you were asked to identify the values that underpin your profession. The use of coercion and force as outlined above are clearly in conflict with such values. It is unlikely that any of you would enter your profession intending to practise in this way. It is not known how those who undertook these acts felt when they set out on their professional journey: they may too have felt the same. The issues that were linked to the abuse within the organisation at Winterbourne View were multi-layered and complex, influenced by national, organisational and professional cultures (Flynn, 2012). Ultimately, these factors may be uncovered because physical abuse is observable, but it took people from the family cultures a long time to get the more dominant organisational cultures to actually see what they saw. Cultural power can be hard to see, even when abuse is visible, and it can be very hard for people who are less powerful to change dominant cultures. Manipulation may be even harder to spot at an organisational or professional level, because it is hidden. Not only is it hidden, but the techniques that are used in manipulation may be closely aligned to those that professionals use routinely when working with service users to support people to undertake activities that are believed to be in their best interests. Best interests tests may be used to judge whether to give people treatment even if they don't want it (DoH, 2005), or to limit their choices if professionals feel that they have reduced capacity to make an informed decision (DoH, 2007). How these issues fit within Lukes' framework is interesting: if the individual does not want that treatment, then the issue becomes conflictual and those in authority may have to use power to achieve their goal. In theory the power therefore is manipulation, but in practice, force may be required to administer treatment. Professionals may use persuasion, encouragement or inducement to support people to do things like lose weight, give up alcohol or support their children more effectively. According to Lukes, these techniques are influence, rather than power, as the interests of the professional and that of the service user do not conflict. When the interests of both parties coincide he argues that power in any form ceases to be an issue. However, this leads us to a very pragmatic problem within Lukes' framework: who decides what constitutes best interests? Can professionals be certain that what they are doing is influencing people to help them achieve their true interests, or are they being manipulated to adhere to the norms that professionals or members of the dominant culture have established? Lukes' third dimension of power has been critiqued for being normatively evaluative (Haugaard, 2002); that is to say, it tends to judge what a best interest is against the norms developed by the more powerful people within a culture.

Within this book, we argue that there is always a power differential within any interaction in health and social care settings when staff and service users interact. Members of an organisation or professional culture have access to the language that frames knowledge, and they have greater access to structures that support or hinder power sharing. Professionals also make judgements according their own norms. Those norms may be developed within a range of cultures as identified in Chapter 1: nationality, ethnicity, gender, class, family, profession and work or social organisations.

We offer the following as a pragmatic solution to the problem of framing best interests when using the model. The professional should consider the problem at hand in relation to the values and norms of a range of the cultures that they personally inhabit. They should then attempt to find the same information from the service user – consider the norms of that person from a range of cultural perspectives. The issue of best interests has then been considered from a multi layered cultural perspective. This sounds complex, but it is the type of decision that we make for ourselves on a daily basis as Box 2.6 illustrates. The issue at hand is not particularly contentious, but the reasoning that went on behind the scenes was discussed with the Communicate2U in the process of writing this book: does the professional provide a healthy snack or unhealthy biscuits to aid the writing process?

The example shows that even simple decisions contain dimensions of power. As the professional, Annette retains the power to make a decision for the rest of the group as she holds the financial and practical resources. These small

The healthy or unhealthy snack dilemma			
Cultural Lens	The professional perspective – Annette (occupational therapist)		Perspective of a service user with a learning disability
National – UK	Mid-morning drink with a snack is a cultural norm	National – UK	Mid-morning drink with a snack is a cultural norm
Ethnicity – English	Tea with a biscuit is normal	Ethnicity – English	Tea with a biscuit is normal
Family	A couple of biscuits at around 11 is normal AND We are a healthy family that likes to stick to a reasonable weight May sometimes have fruit instead	Family	A couple of biscuits around 10.30 is normal AND We are a healthy family that likes to stick to a healthy weight May sometimes have fruit instead
Professional	Should promote healthy eating and lifestyle A shared snack time promotes group cohesion and encourages attendance at the group	Professional	Not applicable
Organisational (health or social care workplace)	Should promote health when in contact with service users (should offer fruit) Costs need to be kept down (biscuits are cheaper) Time is at a premium (biscuits are easier – they last, fruit doesn't)	Organisational	Member of Communicate2U. People with a learning disability should be involved in decision making within the organisation. I should help to make the decision about the snack
Personal decision to be made	Should I offer the group fruit or biscuits? I prefer biscuits (but know I should be eating fruit) I'm not overweight Whose interests do I prioritise – mine, the organisations', or those of the group members?	Personal decision to be made	If a snack is offered, will I take it? I like to have the choice I prefer biscuits (but think this may be on my list of unhealthy things I shouldn't eat) I'm a bit overweight

Box 2.6: Power and best interests – the snack dilemma

decisions may appear unimportant in organisations in which life and death decisions have to be made. However, this level of interaction can form the backdrop against which our values are based, and it is the minutia of daily interactions that can have the biggest influence on people who are otherwise excluded from decision-making processes (Ramcharan, 1997; Ramcharan et al., 2001). We don't all make huge decisions every day, but we often decide on whether to offer snacks or not to visitors. Therefore, it is an opportunity to practise the skills associated with power sharing on a regular basis. As Malcolm illustrates in the quotation, knowledge of cultural norms can be empowering. Malcolm is a teacher who supported service users who had a learning disability and their parents at multi-disciplinary meetings. He became increasingly annoyed at how they were excluded from major decisions that affected their lives. He used his cultural awareness of the impact of the physical act of providing biscuits to force social care staff to enact the social convention of providing drinks in order to help to facilitate communication. Have a go at the exercise in Box 2.7 to help you to understand the hidden power and values that Malcolm was aware of.

And it wasn't (just) ... the language, often, that was used, the sheer fact that in 95% of the meetings, the parents weren't even offered a drink, which is a very simple starter for anybody to do. It made the meetings far more difficult than they needed to be ... It got to the situation where, in one social services office in particular, I used to bring biscuits, which forced them into making tea and coffee so that we could all sit around and at least have a drink. (Malcolm, Communicate2U)

Communicate2U quotation 2.2: Malcolm uses the power of biscuits!

Both Box 2.7 and Malcolm's quotation illustrate the next point in our exploration of power. Power and communication cannot be separated. If you are to understand the norms of another culture, you have to be able to communicate at some level with members of that culture. If you cannot communicate, you will not take into account their cultural norms, and you will make decisions based only on your own cultural knowledge. That means that as a professional, you run the risk of using manipulation (or even professionally sanctioned coercion or force) to achieve your own aims, whilst believing that you are acting in the best interests of the service users with whom you interact. You also run the risk of overlooking situations in which the cultural norm within the family is that of domination or even harming the service user: this experience may be alien to your own cultural expectations and therefore you fail to see it. The next section will consider how the balance between verbal and non-verbal communication used by professionals may affect power relations with service users.

**Professional/
Organisational Lens**

Think about organisations in which you have worked.

? **Which visitors get offered a drink or snack?**

? **Why?**

? **What would happen if an important visitor came to the organisation and was not offered a drink?**

? **What does this say about power?**

? **What does this say about the way in which Malcolm's service users were viewed?**

Box 2.7: The power of a hot drink

The Bacon Butty Song

View this song online to help you remember the three dimensions of power, and the impact that these can have on service users in real life.

A couple of terms that you may be unfamiliar with and that you will need in order to understand the song are:

Bacon butty = bacon sandwich

Caff = café

? Having watched the video, how do you think staff could have dealt with the situation in such a way as to maximise empowerment, whilst still dealing with the issue of limited resources?

? Try to map your response to each of the three dimensions of power.

Box 2.8: The bacon butty song: the three dimensions of power in the real world

Summary of the Three Dimensions of Power

The three dimensions of power may still seem a little abstract to you, but the practical repercussions of this are very evident to service users who are reliant upon staff within their daily lives. When power was discussed with Communicate2U, they could easily give examples of times that they had been disempowered. The example that they chose to share was that of a group home where people had not been allowed to go out as usual to meet their friend Sue for breakfast. The reasons given were linked to a lack of resources, such as money and staffing (first dimension), and that their choice of a bacon sandwich (or butty) was unhealthy (best interests – third dimension). When they suggested ways of reducing costs (such as going by bike instead of a car or taxi), their ideas were ignored (second dimension of agenda and bias). The song that they wrote is a very simple way of remembering and identifying the three dimensions of power. It also demonstrates how creative people can be with their ideas for transport when given an open agenda! Go online and listen to it to help reinforce what you have learned. Then answer the questions posed in Box 2.8.

WORDS AS CULTURAL DOMINATION – A HIDDEN ASPECT OF HEALTH AND SOCIAL CARE

At the end of Chapter 1, you were asked to consider health and social care organisations and professions as examples of low context, technical cultures. In other words, they are cultures in which professional members gain their knowledge through formal education systems. The ability to access the spoken and written word is a fundamental principle of higher education; it is taken for granted, and is therefore a cultural norm that would benefit from closer examination.

Literacy enables people to find out about their world. If this is combined with critical thinking it also enables less dominant people to challenge those in power – it is therefore an incredibly powerful tool (Friere, 1986). Reflective and critical thinking skills are aspects of practice that are embedded within many health and social care courses (Callister et al., 2009; Carr, 2004; Crowe et al., 2006; Higgs et al., 2008; Mattingly et al., 1994). This book is making active use of those skills every time we ask you to undertake the activities in the boxes. So far, so good.

However, whilst many of these foundational principles are excellent, they also carry with them dangers for vulnerable people. Friere (1986), who first advocated them and whose philosophies underpin many educational systems, went on to assert that it is the human capacity to reflect, think, and view knowledge in terms of past and future actions that distinguishes humans from the animals. His definitions of humanity therefore exclude people who lack the capacity for symbolic thought and who cannot communicate by using words. Excluding people from a definition of humanity even in an unintended and unconscious way has serious implications. Cultural norms for dealing with people are based upon this type of definition, and those excluded do not experience the same rights and considerations as the rest of society. The atrocities committed by the Nazi regime upon people who they defined as less than human (such as the Jews, people with some disabilities and gypsies) illustrate this point vividly. Viewing Friere's work in this way means that what was intended as an educational pedagogy for liberating the general population actually may oppress the most vulnerable members of society, who lack the capacity to understand and communicate by using words. The ability to understand and use words is recognised as an explicit power resource by some theorists (Bourdieu, 1991), and is implicit within all three dimensions of power outlined above (Bachrach *et al.*, 1963; Bachrach *et al.*, 1962; Dahl, 1968; Lukes, 1974). Those without the ability to use words are therefore vulnerable to disempowerment within cultures in which words are the dominant form of communication. However, the use of words is so prevalent within many cultures it is a hidden norm and those in a position to dominate and oppress by using them may be not be conscious that they are doing so.

VULNERABLE COMMUNICATORS IN HEALTH AND SOCIAL CARE SETTINGS

This book uses many examples of people with a learning disability (PWLD) as being people who are vulnerable within health and care interactions for a number of reasons. They are a cultural group that have been excluded from definitions of humanity and its consequent rights and responsibilities for many generations (Atkinson *et al.*, 2005; Foucault, 1965; Goodey, 2011; Neugebauer, 1996). Their communication is often framed in terms of the degree to which it varies from the skill base of the general ('normal') population (Mashal *et al.*, 2012; Tager-Flusberg, 1985; Tager-Flusberg *et al.*, 1990; Tager-Flusberg *et al.*, 2009). Since PWLD have often been segregated from society, social inclusion is an ongoing issue within many national cultures (DoH Chang *et al.*, 2007; 2009; Horner-Johnson *et al.*, 2002; Hubert, 2006). Therefore, people in the general population may have had limited opportunity to interact with PWLD to experience communication with this cultural group first hand. Those same people go on to become health and social care professionals. When they meet a service user who has a learning disability they are often fearful of communicating, do not know what to do and are afraid to try (Gibbs *et al.*, 2008; Lachetta *et al.*, 2011; Sowney *et al.*, 2007). Many of the problems that are experienced by PWLD when they interact with health and social care staff are common to other cultural groups that may be set apart from the general population because of their communication styles. Examples of such populations include people with dementia (de Vries, 2013; Eggenberger *et al.*, 2013; Passalacqua *et al.*, 2012; Veselinova, 2014), people with mental health needs (Barnes *et al.*, 2001; Department of Health, 2011; Hatton, 2009; Phillips, 2005), neurological conditions (Balandin *et al.*, 2007b; Coleman *et al.*, 2013; Lancioni *et al.*, 2010; Lancioni *et al.*, 2012; McDermott *et al.*, 2014; Sargent *et al.*, 2013; Stasolla *et al.*, 2013; Togher, 2013) or additional sensory needs (Barnett, 2002b; Bunning *et al.*, 2013; Detaille *et al.*, 2003; Harris, 1995). There are therefore a wide range of service users who may not use words to communicate in the same way as the general population. Staff tend to lack experience and confidence in communicating with people whose cultural styles of communication differ from their own, and all the barriers to effective intercultural communication outlined in Chapter 1 (Barna, 1997) come into play. Difficulties in using word-based communication are not limited to the above groups. People who are part of the 'normal' general population may also experience times when they are unable to use words effectively – for example, if they are intubated (Arif-Rahu *et al.*, 2010; Bard *et al.*, 2004; Tate *et al.*, 2012), anxious or their first language is not that of the dominant culture (Nimmon, 2007; Yip, 2012). However, the vast majority of all of these people listed above will communicate well enough in family or friendship cultural groupings to make their needs understood and to cause those around them to respond. Non-professionals such as family members may have the skills and knowledge to communicate effectively with vulnerable people who find using words hard. Therefore, having a skills deficit in the use of words is not the deciding factor that makes these people communicatively vulnerable in health and social care settings. What makes people vulnerable is staff who lack the ability to change their communication style to one that more closely matches that of the person with whom they are interacting. Health and social care staff can make people vulnerable. People may struggle to understand or use words for a wide variety of reasons and they may hide this lack of understanding if they have the capacity to do so (Goffman, 1959; Goffman, 1963). If staff in health and social care settings fail to notice that the words they are using are not the most effective means of communication, or they notice and do nothing to change their communication style, then they fail to address power imbalances. A failure to address power imbalances during communication exchanges makes people vulnerable. Vulnerable communicators often lack capacity to adapt their way of communicating, but you don't. As a professional, you hold the power. You can decide how the interaction will go, and you can decide how much you will adapt your communication style. You are the person that can make a service user communicatively vulnerable or empowered during the interaction.

A starting point for reducing vulnerability is to define effective communication within health and social care settings in terms that do not refer to words. The definition that is used as the conceptual framework for this book is influence by both Scollen *et al.* (2012) and Bunning *et al.* (2009) and is as follows:

> Effective communication with vulnerable people occurs when the most powerful communicator within an exchange acknowledges and responds to the emotional (and if present, factual) message sent in a manner that is consistent with the cultural style of the least powerful communicator

Communication is therefore an active process and the cultural context in which the interaction occurs is an essential component. The final section within this chapter brings together the issues of power and communication in a diagram to help you to start to map the impact of your communication style upon service users.

MAPPING COMMUNICATIVE VULNERABILITY

Have a look at the simple diagram below that has been developed through research with people with a learning disability, their families, support workers and teachers. It is based upon the following principles:

- Power and communication are interlinked
- Some service users find words hard and prefer other ways of communicating
- Non-word-based communication may be more effective
- Staff who adapt notice power imbalances and make adjustments to their communication style so that they can improve communication with vulnerable people
- Staff who don't notice power imbalances and don't make adjustments to their communication style can harm vulnerable people

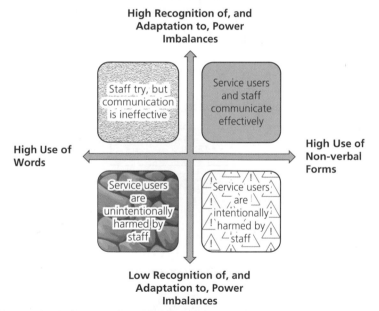

Figure 2.3: Mapping the impact of staff communication strategies on vulnerable service users

You may have noticed that power and communication issues are presented in a similar format to that used in the mixing desk exercises. They are on a spectrum, and in real-life situations, the position that a person adopts may vary greatly during a communication exchange. When considered as a whole (i.e. an average as to the pattern of communication that occurred throughout an exchange), interactions with an individual can be mapped in the following ways:

Effective Communication (The Smooth Zone)

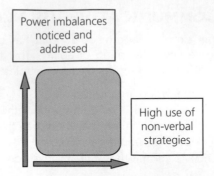

The member of health or social care staff notices that a service user is finding words hard and they adjust their communication style. They include a high degree of non-verbal strategies that try to match the preferred style of the service user. They look to see if these strategies are effective, and if not, adjust again. The service user or their family/carer feel that they have been listened to and are happy with the exchange. Communication occurs smoothly. There is an increased likelihood that the service user's needs will be addressed.

Empowerment in Theory But Not in Practice (The Bumpy Zone)

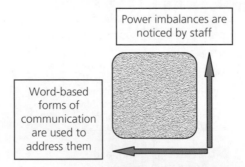

Communication within the bumpy zone is characterised by staff recognising that a service user is struggling with communication, but failing to adjust their communication style effectively. They may try to simplify the language that is used, but still use a lot of words to communicate. Instructions and supporting information provided in words may therefore not be understood by the service user. Staff may ask if the service user has understood, and be satisfied if they respond by saying 'yes'. Communication is ineffective.

Disempowering Communication (The Rocky Zone)

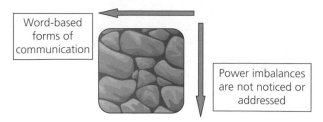

Staff who communicate in the rocky zone do not intend to harm service users. However, they fail to notice that using words may be disempowering. They give information in the form of words and overlook information from the service user that is predominantly non-verbal in nature. They may overlook body language or sounds that indicate distress as they do not see it as communication. This type of communication can result in physical harm, and in extreme cases, the unnecessary deaths of vulnerable service users (Mencap, 2013; Mencap, 2006).

Domination and/or Abuse (The Danger Zone)

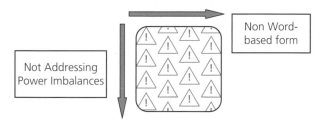

Staff who operate within the danger zone do not address power imbalances and may use physical domination (also a non-verbal form of communication) to communicate with vulnerable people. They cause foreseeable distress and harm. Communication in the Winterbourne serious case review can be classified within this zone (Flynn, 2012).

CHAPTER SUMMARY

As a professional you have tremendous power over service users, even if you think you are at the bottom of the organisational hierarchy. Knowing the forms that this power takes, and the ways in which it is shared (or not), can help you to map how much of this power you share with others. If you fail to do this, you may inadvertently cause harm to the most vulnerable people that you come into contact with in health and social care settings. Using a model to think about how you spot power differentials and adapt communication from verbal to non-verbal formats can help to reduce the risk of you doing this. In the chapters that follow, you will have the opportunity to learn more about how to communicate with vulnerable service users in ways that are empowering.

EASY READ CHAPTER SUMMARY

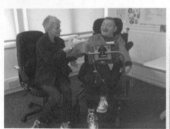 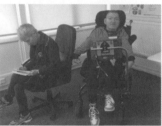

People can choose to share power and the things they know, or keep it to themselves.

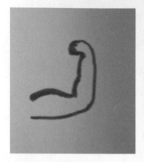 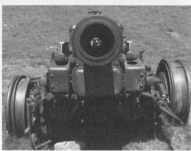

There are lots of different types of power.

Power like guns or strong arms is easy to see.

Other kinds of power are harder to see.

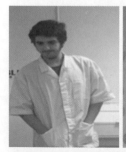 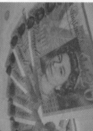 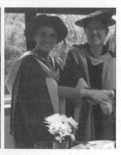

People can have power because they:

- Have a job that others think is important
- Have money
- Know lots of things

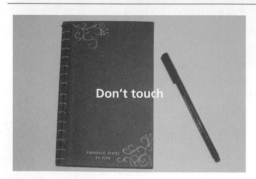

People sometimes write a list of things it's ok to talk about.

This is called an agenda.

Controlling what goes on the list gives people power.

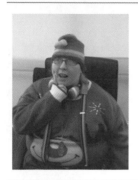

People may think about what is best for others.

This is also part of power.

If they want to share power, they need to value what the other person thinks.

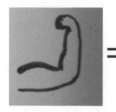 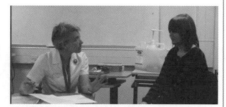

Power is linked to how well people communicate.

It can be hard for some people to use words.

If people find words hard, they often have less power.

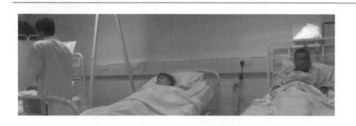

If people like doctors, nurses, therapists or social workers only use words they can hurt people.

They don't mean to do that.

They need to see communication as well as hear it.

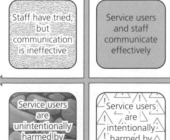 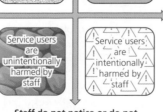

They can use a picture to help them learn to think about power and communication.

This can help them to stop hurting people by mistake.

Word–Based Interpersonal Communication

By the end of this chapter you will be able to:

➡ Describe how the words that you use are linked to your cultural groups

➡ Reflect upon the links between words, power and culture

➡ Identify how health and social care cultures use words to frame interpersonal exchanges with service users

➡ Assess the impact of professional and institutional word-based practices upon the service user experience

Introduction

Chapter 2 started by stating that words are slippery things, and it concluded by arguing that in prioritising word-based communication, staff in health and social care settings have the potential to make service users vulnerable. The subject of words therefore clearly requires closer examination. The question as to how to train health and social care staff to communicate effectively is one that has been the subject of intensive research and review. Communication training includes consideration of both verbal and non-verbal communication (Chant *et al.*, 2002; Eggenberger *et al.*, 2013; Lewin *et al.*, 2001; Perry *et al.*, 2013); therefore, in theory, staff should be in a position to use words to communicate well. However, when service users or carers feel that they have been failed within health and social care settings, their complaints often start with identifying basic communication errors. The causes of such failures are multi-factorial, but the need to change the culture of care to avoid future repetitions is a common theme within the enquiries that have followed (Francis, 2013; Heslop *et al.*, 2013). However, cultural change is not easy, and from discussions in Chapters 1 and 2 you should be aware that existing members of the culture may be those least likely to be in a position to identify what needs to be done (Hall, 1959). This chapter draws upon the experiences of people who may be vulnerable in health and social care communication exchanges and those who work closely with them. Their expertise as communication experts with Communicate2U and within their own family cultures informs the intercultural approach to word-based communication that follows.

By the end of this chapter we will have explored why seemingly innocuous words can have a powerful impact on communication exchanges in a range of cultural settings, and how words have come to be such a powerful component within our lives. This chapter will build upon the issues of culture that were identified in Chapter 1, and the issues of power identified in Chapter 2. It will explore the hidden patterns of cultural communication that determine how we use words. In doing so you will be able to identify how these patterns manifest themselves in health and social care settings, and how your words may affect your service users.

THE CULTURAL CONTEXT OF WORD-BASED COMMUNICATION

Words are such a ubiquitous part of our everyday lives that we often take them for granted. We rarely stop to think about how and why we come to use a particular word in a given situation. If we do, it is often only briefly (for example because the word is unfamiliar to us or we are searching for exactly the right term to use in an important communication). Once the newness and novelty wears off, words become everyday things that fade into the background and their power is hidden. However, words and the way that individuals understand them (or not) are not as obvious as we may first think.

Saussure was a linguist who looked at this issue in some depth. He noted that a spoken word is a purely arbitrary sound (the signifier) that identifies an object or a concept (the signified) to another. Words themselves only have meaning because people who use them have agreed that this is so. The agreed meaning can only be clear if people have knowledge of its use within a culture. What we identify as a 'dog' in English is 'hund' in German and 'cane' in Italian: very different sounds

Words and meaning

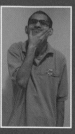

An example of a word that has shifted meaning over time in the English language is the word 'gay'. At the start of the 20th century it denoted a state of happiness, and by the end of the same century it denoted sexual orientation.

A word that has a different meaning in England and America is 'fall'. In addition to being a verb that is understood in both countries, it also denotes a season in America.

Think about films you have watched that either are set in the past or in a different country or region that speaks the same language.

Try to identify as many words as possible that:

? **mean different things in different languages**

? **have a different meaning now to in the past**

How may this impact upon your communication with people from different areas or age groups?

Do we always use words?

Think about the word 'stop'. How many different ways can you think of to show this word? (Thinking of traffic control or trying to stop someone from talking may help you here.) A couple of examples are shown below to start you off...

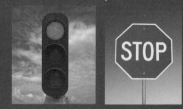

Box 3.1: Words and variety of meaning

that mean the same thing to people from different language systems. Even if we agree on a sound, meanings can shift over time, and the way that a word is pronounced may vary widely between people from different geographical locations (Culler, 1976). Saussure also identified that the use of words to communicate may also be arbitrary – the signifier could equally be a written word, or another form of symbol. The exercise in Box 3.1 illustrates these points.

Thinking about words from a national cultural perspective highlights the arbitrary nature of this form of communication most vividly. People from a Western cultural background may use different words to denote the picture shown below; however, they would all be likely to classify the animal concerned under a wider heading of 'pet' or 'working animal'. They would be unlikely to use the term 'food' to identify a dog, but consumption of dog meat is an accepted norm within many cultures (Jandt, 2007). Later in this chapter we will be exploring examples of how a different meaning attached to words by service users and staff can have far-reaching consequences. For now we will focus on the wider issue of the use of words themselves as a means of communicating, and the hidden values that are connected with this.

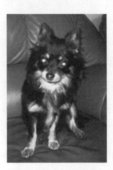

Since we are exploring communication from an intercultural perspective, we will use a cultural model of communication to identify where words are sited within the communication process. The model used was developed by Hymes (2005) who critiqued traditional communication models that were based on two people (sender and receiver of information) as being inadequate. He argued that communication at an interpersonal level is underpinned by the relationship that participants have, which in turn is influenced by cultural determinants. It consists of the following:

Table 3.1: Table illustrating Hymes' (2005) components of communication

The component	What it consists of
The message form	How things are said (e.g. writing, speech, symbols)
Message content	The topic: introduction and maintenance

Table 3.1 *Continued*

Setting	The time, place and physical circumstances surrounding the interaction
Scene	Cultural definitions of the occasion
Participants	Who is involved and their identified roles
Purpose (cultural)	The expected outcome of the interaction from a cultural perspective (e.g. the conventional outcome that may be expected from a health check-up or meeting with a social worker)
Purpose (individual)	The goal that an individual has in relation to an interaction
Key	The tone or manner associated with the interaction (e.g. jokey or serious). This may be in conflict with the overt message content (e.g. when sarcasm is used)
Channels	Written, spoken or oral channels (e.g. oral channels may include humming, singing or chanting)
Form of speech	This is influenced by three criteria: 1. Historical provenance (language and dialect) 2. Mutual intelligibility (codes) 3. Specialisation (technical language)
Norm of interaction	Specific behaviours that are associated with the norms of the interaction (e.g. children are not expected to interrupt a teacher)
Norms of interpretation	How different people may view the event – these particularly relate to the cultural norms that develop within groups

Hymes' (2005) model underpins subsequent chapters in which we explore interactions between health and social care staff and service users. This chapter will focus predominantly on word-based, oral forms of communication. In Chapter 1, we identified that staff in health and social care settings often work in technical, low context cultures. The term **technical** is used to identify that the norms, values and skills associated with professions or organisations have been identified explicitly. This technical knowledge is passed on from expert teachers to novice students by using words in either a verbal or written format. Examples of the ways in which technical knowledge is imparted include lectures, journal articles or books. This type of knowledge transmission is often associated with logical analysis and a defined structure. It has been consciously learned,

Learning under cultural lenses

Think about how you learn in different cultures to which you belong. Fill in the table below.

Put a tick in the box if the statement applies, and a cross if it doesn't.

	Professional Lens		Social Group Lens
	Learning at university/ college	*Learning on placement*	*Learning to be a friend with a new person*
Explicitly uses research based on written articles/books			
Taught by a person acknowledged to be an expert in the subject			
Factual knowledge is important			
Showing emotion is important			
Knowledge tested in a written format			
Knowledge tested through experience			
The expected ways of behaving are made clear			
Mistakes are clearly identified as soon as they occur			
Consequences of mistakes can be disastrous to others or self			

Box 3.2: How you learn as a professional and with friends

and therefore can be written down and recorded, using technical language, the meaning of which is agreed by respected members of the culture (Hall, 1959). Health and social care professions and organisations have a strong cultural tendency to use and value words as their message form, and the channels used may be both written and oral. Precision in the use of technical language is important since it enables complex information to be transmitted relatively rapidly, with limited or no emotion, and with a reduced risk of misunderstanding between users (Devito, 1997). Anybody who has ever had to pass an exam to become a health and social care professional can tell you how important it is to know the right words and to use them in the right way. There is a cultural norm that requires staff to communicate their message effectively and concisely. However, this type of precision learning has its limitations, and learning also takes place between mentors and students in a **formal** way – the teacher showing and correcting the learner. An example of this would be the type of learning that occurs on placement. The purpose of placement is (amongst other aims) to induct the learner into the norms of the profession, whilst also inducting the learner into the way in which those norms are applied within in a specific setting. Formal learning has a tendency to include practices that may have drifted from the science-based, technical origins. These local cultural norms then become part of the accepted organisational culture. The 'this is the way that we do it' norm is no longer underpinned by explicit and technical knowledge; it is based on hidden formal knowledge that is rarely questioned (Hall, 1959). Have a go at filling in the table in Box 3.2 to identify the role that word-based learning plays in your professional role and compare this to how you learn from friends.

There are several dangers present in health and social care settings if the cultural ways in which word-based communication is learned are not recognised:

- There is a danger that the technical meaning that an individual member of staff associates with a word may differ from the meaning that lay people, or other professionals attach to it.
- There is a danger that the current usage of a word (or the practices associated with it) may have drifted from the original meaning and intent that was culturally agreed.
- There is a danger that non-word-based communication from service users, family or carers may not be valued or may be overlooked.
- There is a danger that some of the non-word-based, emotional learning that occurs within practice may not be valued by staff if it does not occur in an academic, technical context (such as a formal reflection).

To address these potential dangers, it is important that the hidden cultural aspects of word-based communication in health and social care settings are examined more closely since words are the means by which societal knowledge is transmitted across distances and time (Berger *et al.*, 1969).

Words will be considered within the context of the patterns or scripts in which they occur, and then we will focus more closely upon the power that words may have to shape interactions.

AN INTRODUCTION TO SCRIPTING

When people meet in face to face interactions, the encounters are framed by the roles in which the participants are cast, the outcomes that each participant expects the interaction to lead to, and the relative status of participants (Danziger,

1976; Hymes, 2005). Interactions are therefore not quite as unstructured as we may think, and can be viewed as variations or improvisations that are based on existing scripts (Goffman, 1967; Goffman, 1959). Knowing this can help us to analyse what is happening and improve our performances. This chapter will be looking at the words used. It is however important to remember that they are a small component of the overall message, and that they link with other components of the performance such as the musical aspects of speech, body language and the environmental setting. Table 3.2 shows you where these aspects are considered within this book. Culture (Chapter 1) and power (Chapter 2) underpin all of these concepts and so are not shown separately.

Table 3.2: How chapters link within this book: Chapter 3

Chapter 3: Words and how they are used	Chapter 4: How words are said (plus the musical aspects of speech)	Chapter 5: Communicating without words (body language)	Chapter 6: The setting for communication (environmental aspects of communication)	Chapter 7: Putting it all together – performing health and social care scripts

Scripting may sound a little far-fetched, but it is present in even simple day to day interactions. For example, if you approach a stranger to ask them for directions, you do so because you cast them in the role of a person with local knowledge. You hope that the outcome of the interaction is getting the information that you need to find your way. The words that you use to ask for directions may vary depending on how you perceive their status. For example, a young person who is dressed informally (*Hi – any idea where the post office is?*) may be approached in a very different manner to a police officer (*Excuse me, please could you give me directions to the post office?*). Even the simplest of encounters are associated with set patterns – scripts – which the participants either adhere to or manipulate if they think this will give them a better outcome (Danziger, 1976). Scripts can help us to manage the way in which we present ourselves to others to help maintain a good image or 'face' (Goffman, 1959) and they can also serve to speed up the flow of conversation since each person knows what is expected of them from the context of the encounter. However, scripts are developed within cultures, and 'normal' interactions can quickly become complex and fraught with misunderstandings if people come from different cultural backgrounds (Jandt, 2007). When we meet somebody, we unconsciously expect them to adhere to our own scripted pattern, and if they deviate from this, we often view them as rude, ignorant or uncooperative (Scollon *et al.*, 2012). We take on a stance of cultural superiority: they are not conforming to our rules and are therefore the ones who are wrong (Barna, 1997). We don't have to change our behaviour – they do. Only 'they' are often thinking the same thing. The cycle can be difficult to break unless one of the participants recognises that there may be a cultural barrier to communication (Edelstein *et al.*, 1989). Once one person in the encounter starts to view things from an intercultural perspective, the barriers to intercultural communication that were identified in Chapter 1 (Barna, 1997) can be addressed.

Face to face encounters in health and social care are highly scripted. Professional training includes induction into the role that the person is expected to play, the outcomes that they are expected to achieve, and how these should be accomplished in accordance with professional and organisational constraints. Service users on the other hand are likely to have learned their role in an informal manner, based on emotionally charged experiences (see Chapter 1). In order to be effective, practitioners need cultural awareness at many different levels (Bischoff *et al.*, 2014). They need to be aware of their own cultural communication scripts, those of the organisations with which they interact, and also (most importantly) the scripts adopted by the service users. This chapter focuses on words. We will examine the words associated with roles in health and social care settings, and the impact that these have upon the way in which scripts are played out.

ROLES IN HEALTH AND SOCIAL CARE

The general expectations of an interaction are established long before participants actually meet face to face in a health or social care setting (Danziger, 1976). The majority of service users and carers will have developed an informal internal image of how they expect the named professional to act. This may be based on previous encounters with health or social care staff, or on other models that they have seen (for example on the TV). The word associated with your profession is therefore powerful all by itself. In Chapter 1, we examined how cultural heroes can be used to help identify professional values, and most scripts need both villains as well as heroes. In preparation for the next section, have an honest attempt at the exercise in Box 3.3 because, however unfair it may seem, you will appear as both hero/heroine and villain during your professional career. This may be because

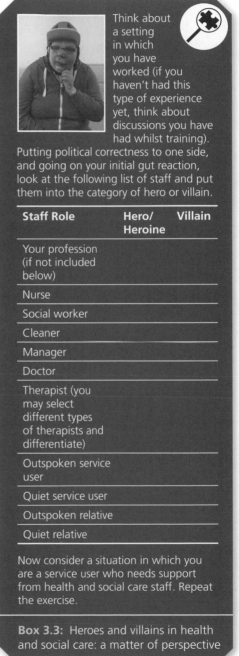

Think about a setting in which you have worked (if you haven't had this type of experience yet, think about discussions you have had whilst training). Putting political correctness to one side, and going on your initial gut reaction, look at the following list of staff and put them into the category of hero or villain.

Staff Role	Hero/ Heroine	Villain
Your profession (if not included below)		
Nurse		
Social worker		
Cleaner		
Manager		
Doctor		
Therapist (you may select different types of therapists and differentiate)		
Outspoken service user		
Quiet service user		
Outspoken relative		
Quiet relative		

Now consider a situation in which you are a service user who needs support from health and social care staff. Repeat the exercise.

Box 3.3: Heroes and villains in health and social care: a matter of perspective of the actions that you take when interacting with service users, or it may be because others in your profession have already set the scene and service users or carers expect you to enact the role in the same way.

Words associated with roles are not neutral collections of sounds. They are the means by which relationships are defined (Danziger, 1976) and socio-cultural norms are acted out (Kiesling, 2005). Within the introduction to this book, the thorny topic of what to call people who receive services from health and social care staff was considered at length for good reason. Labelling theory has identified that the more powerful individual has the potential to use words to define others in ways that disadvantage them (Hirschi, 1975; Scheff, 1974). Chapter 2 identified that all staff in health and social care settings carry a considerable amount of power. This includes the power to decide what to call people who engage with us, and what value and meaning is attached to those words. From an intercultural perspective, the issue of role names becomes more complex since the meaning of words may be very localised. For example, whilst at a national cultural level a word such as patient may be understood by all to indicate a person who is in receipt of medical intervention, at the organisational or professional level of culture the way in which a patient is expected to behave may differ greatly. Within the UK, for example, there has been a shift in emphasis from the notion of a patient as being a passive recipient of care provided by experts (Parsons, 1951) to that of an active participant in the decision-making process (DoH, 2006). The terms that are associated with such a change include words such as 'service user', 'client', 'customer', 'consumer' or 'expert patient'. The shift in terminology is associated with an expectation that the person thus labelled will take on more responsibility to define and achieve set goals (Taylor Gooby, 2008b). However, changing the word by which a person's role is defined does not automatically change the way in which they view themselves, or the way in which they are viewed by staff (Price, 2013). In Chapter 2 (Box 2.1) you learned how confusing this was for Jeff, who had a learning disability. An individual labelled as a service user who in theory is encouraged to act as a consumer may actually be unfamiliar with this role or may wish for more experienced professionals to make decisions on their behalf (Cameron, 2013; Taylor Gooby, 2008a). A member of staff who uses the term service user may in fact be more familiar and comfortable with being viewed as an expert who defines the way in which the interaction occurs (Price, 2013). Even within the same organisation, different professionals may use different words to define the person for whom they provide a service, and the person on the receiving end may prefer to be defined by a different word entirely, for example 'survivor' or 'user by experience' (McLaughlin, 2009; Simmons et al., 2010). When professionals and service users have different views as to how they should play their roles, the result is often unsatisfactory for both parties. Staff may view service users as uncooperative or challenging and may attempt to minimise their contact with the difficult person, thus providing a decreased level of care. Service users or carers may view staff in the same light, increasing the risk of complaints or litigation (Price, 2013).

The definition of a service user as an individual who takes on some responsibility within the decision-making process may make it difficult for staff to view people who have alternative forms of communication as partners within interactions. When service users do not use words to communicate in a formal manner, they fail to conform to the imaged script that staff have in place. For example, they may seem to lack the skills to engage in the typical word-based information exchange that is implicitly associated with the joint planning of goals. People who lack a formal symbolic system for communicating, such as people with late stage dementia (Price, 2013) or a severe learning disability (Mencap, 2013; Mencap, 2006), may be overlooked entirely as a communication partner at all stages of an interaction, from the greeting onwards. Problems with role definition may also occur in settings in which staff and service users have prolonged contact, such as in care homes. In such cases, the role of the professional may need modification from the definition that they may use in a different setting for short-term interactions. Short-term interactions are often characterised by a formal distancing between staff and service users as there is limited opportunity to get to know people better and a pressure on time to complete tasks. This type of role feels too formal and unfriendly in settings where there is prolonged contact. Staff may attempt to redefine their role with service users to one that is less formal, such as 'friend' (Antaki *et al.*, 2007b). Role expectations are therefore closely linked with the type of distance that staff maintain when engaging with those that they care for, and with the communication strategies that they use to manage their interpersonal interactions (Lernihan *et al.*, 2010).

At this point, it is important for you to define what words you use to define health and social care roles and what your expectations of these words are. At a theoretical level, for example, you may use the word service user and associated terms such as person-centred care. On a day to day basis, however, you may actually prefer the person to let you take the lead during key points of the interaction. We will use the concept of heroes and villains to help you to examine the hidden aspects of culture that underpin the values. Have a go at the exercise in Box 3.4 to help you understand how your hidden role expectations may affect the way in which you interact with service users.

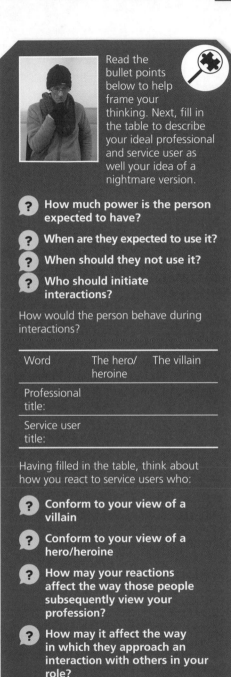

Read the bullet points below to help frame your thinking. Next, fill in the table to describe your ideal professional and service user as well your idea of a nightmare version.

? How much power is the person expected to have?

? When are they expected to use it?

? When should they not use it?

? Who should initiate interactions?

How would the person behave during interactions?

Word	The hero/ heroine	The villain
Professional title:		
Service user title:		

Having filled in the table, think about how you react to service users who:

? Conform to your view of a villain

? Conform to your view of a hero/heroine

? How may your reactions affect the way those people subsequently view your profession?

? How may it affect the way in which they approach an interaction with others in your role?

Box 3.4: Heroes/heroines and villains: how role scripting affects interactions with service users

Given all the confusion listed above, it may be tempting to give up on the idea of examining the words associated with roles at this point. However, from an intercultural perspective, the key points to remember are:

1. The words that you use to define yourself as a professional and the words you use to define people you work with carry values and meaning
2. The values and meaning that you hold in theory may differ when you are actually in practical situations
3. The values and meaning that you associate with these words may differ from those of other people
4. The values and meaning associated with the words may vary at different cultural levels – for example, at the national level, professional level, organisational level and family level
5. If you assume that other people have your understanding of the words, you are setting the scene for a clash of cultures

Understanding that others may hold different assumptions with regards to roles and scripts is a key first step in minimising the risk of inter culturalclashes (Barna, 1997). Danziger (1976) notes that all interpersonal interactions are, at the most basic level, scenarios in which the participants attempt to define their roles in relation to one another in order to achieve their desired outcomes for the interaction. The next section will therefore focus on what professionals and service users may expect to gain from their interactions with each other, and how they frame this.

OUTCOMES OF HEALTH AND SOCIAL CARE INTERACTIONS

Verbal communication occurs because at least one of the participants in an exchange has an underlying purpose that they wish to achieve. Purposes (and their associated outcomes) are linked to both individual and cultural factors. They are based upon social norms and may consist of both an overt message that is explicit and obvious (factual), and a covert or pragmatic element that is less obvious (emotional) (Danziger, 1976). Taking our earlier example of asking for directions, the overt message (that of finding the post office) is relatively obvious, but there may also have been an underlying need for reassurance (the person was pretty sure that they knew the way, but needed to hear it from someone else). For the outcome to be achieved, there usually needs to be some cooperation between participants (Goffman, 1967). However, if participants have different ideas about the purpose of an exchange, it is less likely to be achieved. Within health and social care settings, exchanges between staff and service users often occur in set patterns to achieve goals that are determined by service priorities. In health and social care interactions, exchanges may broadly be categorised as:

1. Being orientated to achieving a practical task, or
2. Developing the social/emotional relationship between the professional and service user.

This links back to Chapter 1, where we identified that cultures can tend towards high context (the message is explicit and factual or practical) or low context (the message is based on context/working towards maintaining emotional harmony). Words associated with achieving practical tasks include: asking, interviewing, counselling, motivating, educating, problem solving. Those associated with socio-emotional development include terms such as: rapport building and translating (from professional terminology) (Roter *et al.*, 2002). We argue here that staff in health and social care cultures often have time-driven practical outcomes that underpin even emotionally based exchanges (Carpiac-Claver *et al.*, 2007; Ong *et al.*, 2000). Therefore, even when the focus of the interaction is relationship building, it is often the professional that determines what element of the relationship is focused upon, and how much time is invested in this process. This is the norm that has developed within health and social care settings over decades. However, the old cultural norms are gradually changing as service users are expected to take on a more proactive role in their care. This can lead to difficulties on both sides as neither service user nor staff member can be certain as to how to behave whilst the roles and outcomes differ from service to service, and person to person (Taylor Gooby, 2008b). Different expectations with regards to the outcome of exchanges can lead to a culture clash, and this is turn can lead to service user dissatisfaction.

In Chapter 1 we defined culture as being a verb (Scollon *et al.*, 2012). One of the ways in which staff can start to become aware of the degree to which they focus interactions to achieve their own professional or organisational outcome is to examine the types of things that they do. Verbs can be used to explore which person in an interpersonal exchange is taking the lead, or initiating the exchange (Osgood, 1970). Take a look at Box 3.5 below in which some of the words associated with the person actively taking the lead (initiating) and those associated with the person who is more passively responding (or reacting) are listed. Use the exercises and the film produced by Communicate2U to consider how health and social care roles are generally scripted to give more of the active aspects of communication to the staff member.

The outcome that the professional may wish to achieve may well be determined by the way in which the professional views the role of the service user. Where the person in receipt of services is viewed as a patient being treated by a professional then the goal may be to achieve compliance with the most effective intervention. Where the service user is viewed as a partner, the professional goal may that of concordance – coming to a mutually agreed aim (Bissell *et al.*, 2004; Segal, 2007). The outcome of an interaction will, however, be influenced by the setting and social norms associated with the exchange. For example, in ward rounds or case reviews where there is a lot of factual information to be exchanged, service users may be dominated by professionals and be in a position in which their predominant style of communication is that of reaction (Shattell, 2004; Weber *et al.*, 2007). This may make reviews shorter, but the ultimate goal of the exchange – namely to agree a plan that will be carried out in practice by the service user – may not be achieved. Reactive acceptance during the formal meeting may be followed by the service user refuting the professionally dominated agreed outcome. Communication partners have

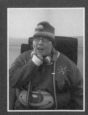

1. Think about the typical exchanges that you as a professional will have with service users or their carers.

List the exchanges and next to each write down the expected outcome for the exchange and guess at the percentage of time in which the service user is in a position to initiate part of the interaction.

An example from an acute therapy setting is given below:

Initial interview (gain baseline background information): 20%

Formal assessment (assess cognitive and perceptual level of functioning): 15%

Practical intervention (work with service user to set goals for intervention and work on improving function): 35%

Informal meeting in corridor (respond to service user concerns about managing at home): 80%

Discharge meeting (discuss care plan for discharge with service user, family and multi-disciplinary team): 15%

2. Consider the outcomes that you hoped to achieve for the exchanges. Now imagine that you are the service user.
   • What would you want the outcomes and percentages to be?
   • How do you think the professional could achieve this?

3. Visit the companion website and watch the video about interactions between professionals and service users. Do the following:

   • Use the verbs listed below to describe the actions of the professional
   • List the verbs that describe the actions of the service user
   • Describe what you think the anticipated outcome of the interaction is
   • Discuss how you think the service user could have had a greater role in initiating elements of the interaction

Initiating (Active)	Reacting (Passive)
• Inspire	• Accept
• Request	• Answer
• Question	• Follow
• Encourage	• Refute
• Guide	
• Compel	
• Provoke	
• Reassure	

Box 3.5: Expected outcomes for health and social care exchanges linked to service user and professional roles and communication styles

a choice as to whether to collaborate with roles and outcomes during inter-actions, or to resist them overtly or covertly (Goffman, 1967). The quotation below illustrates what may happen when there is a discrepancy between how a professional views the role of a service user and how the service user and family view that role. It also shows what can happen when a professional wishes an interaction to focus upon a factual/practical outcome, whilst the service user or carer focus is on the emotional outcome.

Sadie has taken her son (who has a learning disability but who can speak fluently) to the doctor and clearly views him as the person with whom the professional should communicate. She wants her son to be recognised as a valued person who has the right to determine his own health outcomes. Despite her best efforts to ensure that this occurs, the doctor resists seeing her son in this role, instead preferring to pass factual information on to his carer.

> *If the appointment was regarding my son I would always make him sit down in the chair because the appointment is about him. So I would say to my son, 'You sit there with the doctor so you can talk to the doctor,' and I would stand. But he would be facing the doctor so he would literally ... my son would be on eye level with the doctor, the doctor would be looking up to me, over his head, around to wherever I was standing, totally ignoring my son. Yet the appointment is about him. (Sadie)*

Communicate2U quotation 3.1: Sadie's son being ignored as a communication partner

Years later, both Sadie and her son remembered this exchange and still felt angry about it. Whilst the scene described takes place in a doctor's surgery, Communicate2U members described similar scenes occurring with a wide range of professionals in both health and social care settings. Different expectations of roles and outcomes lead to feelings of anger and exclusion for many service users within the company.

We argue here that professionals do not set out to dominate or exclude service users from interpersonal exchanges. However, the professional and organisational drivers under which staff operate tend towards a focus on factual/practical exchanges. Resources are limited and dealing with an emotional agenda can be time consuming. However, a failure to deal with the outcome that a service user or family member expects from an exchange can have far reaching consequences that include a failure to achieve the optimal outcome of care. The outcome that each person in the exchange wishes to achieve will be influenced by a range of cultural lenses. There are ethnic or national expectations as to what health and social care staff should be aiming for; professional and organisational lenses that acknowledge service priorities and family lenses that frame how professionals are viewed. Recognising that your professional expectations of outcomes may differ from those of service users can help to frame the interaction in such a way that misunderstandings are minimised. One of the simplest ways to achieve this is to ask the person to tell or show you what they'd like to gain from their time with you. That way, you know what their agenda is and can acknowledge or address this during your time together. If you fail to do so, you run the risk of exposing your service users to the kind of power biases that Tony experienced in Chapter 2 (Box 2.4). Focusing only on what you want to achieve may mean that you are considered to be a poor professional, and whatever your intended outcome, it will be harder to achieve. To summarise:

1. From an intercultural perspective, the outcome that the professional or organisation may wish to achieve from an interaction may be different to that of the service user or family member
2. The professional often controls the exchange and determines when and how the service user will interact
3. As a professional with intercultural knowledge, it is important to be aware of the outcomes that your profession and organisation wish to achieve within different types of interactions
4. Professional and organisational priorities should be balanced with the outcomes that the service user wishes to achieve
5. Professional and service user outcomes are linked to power, particularly the form of power associated with bias and agendas (see Chapter 2)

The following sections will review key points that occur in word-based exchanges from an intercultural perspective to examine how intercultural misunderstandings can be reduced in order to increase the likelihood of both professional and service user goals being achieved.

Patterned Interactions During Verbal Communication

Communication is governed by unwritten rules that are culturally determined. These rules may help interactions if both parties are familiar with them, but may hinder effective communication if there are different expectations. By recognising some of the underlying patterns that underpin exchanges, staff can be alert to ways in which they may be excluding service users from communication.

Exclusive and Inclusive Communication

Some of the hidden rules revolve around the type of words that are used. During verbal communication, talk may be considered to be inclusive or exclusive. Exclusive talk occurs when the language used prevents everyone present from fully understanding and participating in the exchange. It may occur without those who are excluding others being aware of it, and it may also occur deliberately so that covert communication can take place. By contrast, inclusive talk is accessible to some degree to all present (Devito, 1997). Have a look at Table 3.3 for examples of **inclusive** and **exclusive communication** under different cultural lenses.

In all of the exchanges shown, exclusive communication resulted in a power imbalance between participants. Sometimes that use of power was intentional – in the latter two examples exclusive communication was consciously used. The sisters used the power for their own interests, whilst the staff used the power to protect both the family and organisation. Where the use of exclusive

Table 3.3: Examples of inclusive and exclusive communication in different cultural settings

National Lens: A group of travellers meet in a hostel. The group start discussing their experiences using English as a common tongue. Some members of the group who speak only a few words of English feel excluded, but nod and smile during the conversation when others appear to do so.	English speakers unintentionally exclude non-English speakers Non-English speakers hide their lack of understanding to save embarrassment
Professional Lens: At a case review meeting, a professional explains their intervention and recommendations. They use the terms that they have learned during their studies. A social worker refers to a ward. The nurse nods in understanding. The social worker is referring to a ward of court (a person who has legally been placed under formal protection), the nurse hears the word and thinks of a hospital ward (a room with beds for patients). The meeting continues and the misunderstanding remains hidden.	Professionals use seemingly simple words in their discussion, but the meaning that each profession attaches to these is different. All present believe that they are using inclusive communication, but the confusion over terminology means that talk is exclusive.
Organisational Lens: At a discharge meeting there is some disagreement between hospital staff, social workers and family members. Professional staff are in dispute about which organisation should fund care once the patient is discharged, but do not wish to concern the family who are determined that a particular care home should be used. They start to use abbreviations and acronyms to explore the topic in front of relatives, and then revert to lay language to explain their decision once they come to agreement.	Professional staff intentionally use exclusive language to prevent the family from experiencing undue concern (protecting others). In doing so, they also protect the financial concerns of the organisation (protecting self).
Family Lens: Two older sisters use complex words and abbreviations to discuss their boyfriends in front of their annoying younger brother. When he asks what they're talking about, they say he's too young to understand.	Family members intentionally use exclusive communication to demonstrate their (perceived!) relative maturity (protecting self).

communication was the end result was still that of a disempowered participant within the communication exchange.

Health and social care professionals are regularly confronted with situations in which they have information that they may choose to share with service users, or to withhold. They have to decide how much to share, and what form that sharing will take. As a starting principle, we argue that staff need to share information that affects a service user with the service user themselves, and that they need to do so in a way that is inclusive. We also argue that currently they are likely to use words as their preferred form of information sharing. The reasons for this and the implications of this hidden cultural norm are explored below.

USING WORDS – A HIDDEN CULTURAL NORM

A fair proportion of professional training will consist of teaching those who wish to graduate which words to use if they are to be inducted into the profession. Another part of the training will then consist of telling students when not to use the words that they have just learned. Communication training for health and social care staff often includes advice on how to avoid the use of complex technical language (Chant *et al.*, 2002; Dougherty *et al.*, 2011; Eggenberger *et al.*, 2013), but it is harder to spot the pitfalls in seemingly simple, everyday words. If inclusive communication is the goal, then health and social care professionals also need to recognise that many of their words are used in ways that have been developed in a professional and organisational culture. Have a look at the jargon wheel in Figure 3.1 (which is based on British use of English) to see how professionals from different backgrounds may use a simple word such as 'service'.

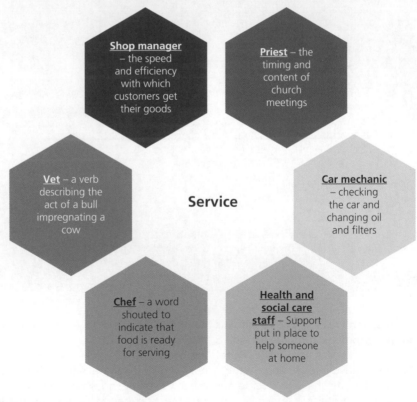

Figure 3.1: The jargon wheel

Professional language can therefore be considered to consist of overt jargon (that is generally easy to spot), and hidden jargon (which is not). When people find using words hard, or they are stressed, they often only pick up on key words within a sentence and may miss other words that contain contextual information that could help to explain the meaning intended (Bild, 2010; Stewart *et al.*, 1999). As a rule of thumb, if a word can have more than one meaning, there is the potential for that word to be misunderstood. Words are interpreted in terms of both formal education and past experiences (Hymes, 2005). Some of the words that you use as a professional may be ones that were previously familiar to you in other cultural settings (such as family or hobby groups). Have a go at the exercise in Box 3.6 to see if you can spot some words that are commonly used in your profession that may be hidden jargon.

Misunderstandings over key words can have a devastating impact on service users. For example, a professional may use the term 'service' to suggest some support to enable daily tasks to be done more easily at home. A service user may have heard the term on the news in connection with social services taking someone into care. The resultant rise in anxiety levels may hinder communication during the rest of the exchange. Clarity over the meaning of words and considering the context of communication are therefore important. Conversations are generally designed in such a way as to give participants clues as to which meaning is being used. The strategies that staff are encouraged to use to enhance communication include:

Having looked at the jargon wheel, have a go at thinking of alternative meanings that could be ascribed to the simple words shown below:

Word	Person using it
Bay	Health or social care staff
	Car mechanic
	Seaside vendor
	Horse breeder
	Botanist
Ward	Health staff
	Solicitor
Care	Nurse
	Social worker
	Family member

Think of your own profession and make a list of words that are :
1. Overt jargon
2. Hidden jargon

Box 3.6: Jargon: same word with different meanings

- Introducing the topic explicitly (giving some context)
- Using non-technical language
- Feeding forward (letting people know what is coming next)
- Chunking information into manageable sizes
- Recapping (telling people what they have been told)
- Summarising
- Attending to feedback that may indicate that the other person has misunderstood (this includes non-verbal aspects of speech such as body language)

(Devito, 1997; Dougherty *et al.*, 2011)

However, all but one of the above elements (feedback) tend to focus on verbal strategies, and therefore vulnerable communicators who find words hard may still not benefit. Nobody likes to admit that they do not understand, and vulnerable

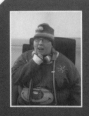 Vicki asked her mum for a tablet. Her mum told her she couldn't have one as they are too expensive. She told her mum that they aren't – you can get them from the chemist!

 or ?

Communiate2U identified some of the words that staff use that can be confusing and Vicki put these into a poem:

Bay

Bay is at the seaside

Bay is a space

Bay is a colour

Bay is a place

Services

Services are workers

Services are for cars

Services are for travellers

When they have driven far

When you interact with others, remember the different meanings that even seemingly simple words can have. This can cause a lot of confusion. Show a picture, act it out, or check we have understood.

Vicki is a performance poet who has written a very powerful poem about the impact of the words associated with labels on her life.

Box 3.7: Communicate2U – same words have different meanings for us and this is confusing

communicators will often have a whole range of strategies in place to make it look as though they have understood (Goffman, 1963). If you as a professional ask someone with these strategies if they have understood, they will say 'yes'. You will think you have communicated, but you could have sown the seeds for misunderstandings at best, and a future disaster at worst.

ALTERNATIVES TO WORDS

Ultimately, words are only symbols that we use for convenience to convey our ideas, and as discussed above, professionals find it very convenient to use words. However, as humans we could equally use other forms of symbolic language to convey our thoughts and wishes to others: sign language, Braille, or a standardised system of whistling – all of these are forms of non-verbal symbolic language that are used within other cultural groups (Jandt, 2007). If professionals limit their symbolic language to one that is for their convenience, rather than that of the service user, then they run the risk of excluding the very people that they wish to support. The trick is to find a symbolic system that is accessible to as many cultural groups as possible.

Pictures and objects have the advantage of being (generally) less abstract than words and they are therefore a lot more accessible. Outside of our professional roles, within our family and social cultural groups, we live in worlds that are dominated not by words, but by images. TV, tablets and phones with their icons, and advertising hoardings with their pictures are all shouting messages to us in ways that are predominantly non-verbal. This is our non-professional world, and that of many service users who find words hard. Visual images that are carefully chosen can cut across cultural boundaries, provide a common language and reduce misunderstandings. Whilst the phrase 'Go to the bay' may be interpreted in a variety of ways, it becomes a lot clearer and less ambiguous when combined with a picture:

'Go to the bay'	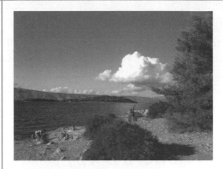
'Go to the bay'	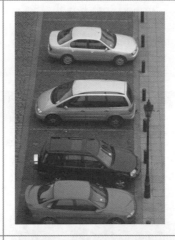
'Go to the bay'	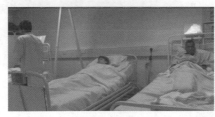

The use of pictures as an adjunct to words is recommended good practice and one that can support people who are otherwise excluded from exchanges to participate (Balandin *et al.*, 2007a; Danielsson *et al.*, 2006; Hemsley *et al.*, 2011; Hemsley *et al.*, 2001; Maginess, 2010; Stephenson *et al.*, 1996; Stoner *et al.*, 2006). It does not have to be limited to formal photographs or symbols – nearly every professional who is required to interact with people has access to a pen and paper. It can take a few moments to do a quick stick drawing, and several minutes to correct a verbal misunderstanding. Books of pictures are available commercially to support communication in a wide range of settings, and free mobile phone apps provide quick and easy access to themed banks of photo-graphs. Yet the majority of exchanges in health and social care settings do not include this type of communicative practice as a cultural norm. The chapter summaries are written in accessible formats:

- Pictures to the left to emphasise their importance
- Short sentences, trying to avoid both covert and overt jargon
- A mixture of lower and upper case letters
- Limit the message to the key points

Think of these principles when you look at Box 3.8 and do the exercises in it.

CHAPTER SUMMARY

This chapter has argued that health and social care staff are culturally primed to use words as the dominant form of communication. Being in charge of the means of communication gives staff hidden power, but that power may not suit

Take a moment to think about times that you have been in practice, on placement, or in a health or social care setting as a service user.

? **How often have you seen pictures used naturally alongside words?**

? **If you have seen this used, what settings did this occur in and what effect did it have?**

? **If you have not seen it used, can you think of situations where it could have been helpful?**

? **If it could have been helpful but wasn't used – what do you think stopped the professional?**

We are more familiar with our roles and what we do in them than service users. The term 'nurse' for example encompasses an enormous variety of job descriptions. We know which one we mean – the service user may be thinking of a past experience with an entirely different type of nurse. To practise getting into the role of a good intercultural communicator, have a go at translating some of your work scripts into a more accessible format.

Think of someone that you know who may find your words hard to understand. This may be a young child or someone who does not have a good grasp of your first language. Alternatively, practise with a tolerant friend!

1. Explain your professional role to them. Don't just use words – use images or objects/actions to supplement these.

2. Explain what you want to achieve from one of your common professional assessments. Again, use images/objects or actions as well as words.

Initially, you will probably find this uncomfortable and embarrassing as it is outside your normal professional script.

Get used to it! You need this skill to communicate well with vulnerable people.

Box 3.8: Using a mixture of words and visual communication to make things easier to understand service users who now expect to have a more active role and say in their care. Words can be ambiguous at best, and at worst can exclude the most vulnerable communicators. This can cause negative feelings with service users and carers. Recognising that the use of words is culturally patterned can help staff to critically evaluate how they communicate at a professional and organisational level. They can then start to adapt their communication and try to routinely include adjuncts to words, such as pictures, objects and signs, so that they don't inadvertently exclude people who find it hard to understand, but don't like to admit this.

EASY READ CHAPTER SUMMARY

	Staff often only use words when they talk to service users
	Some people find words hard to understand
	If there are lots of words, some people can be left out
 Assessment Finding things out	Staff need to use the kind of words we all use – not hard words

Which plaster do they mean?

Plaster on the wall?

This kind of plaster?

This kind of plaster?

Words can mean more than one thing

Staff also need to use pictures

Then we'll know which one they mean

The word plaster can mean lots of things

If staff show us real things as they talk, this can make it easier to understand

Or they can use actions to show us what they really mean

THE MUSICAL ASPECTS OF COMMUNICATION

Aims

By the end of this chapter you will be able to:

➡ Identify what the musical aspects of speech are

➡ Explain why and how musical aspects of speech affect communication

➡ Reflect upon your own musical style of communication

➡ Critically evaluate the impact of different musical communication styles upon interactions between staff and service users

INTRODUCTION

Chapter 3 focused upon the kinds of words that staff and service users use. This chapter will focus upon how those words are said, and how people who don't use words at all may still use sounds to communicate. There are technical terms such as **prosody** or **paralanguage** that we could have used within the title for this chapter. They refer to the non-verbal elements of speech such as pitch, tone, timing and pace of speech, but the terms are often used to focus upon the deficiencies of people who find words difficult (Ayotte *et al.*, 2002; Diehl *et al.*, 2008; Eigsti *et al.*, 2011; Huss *et al.*, 2011; Lim, 2010; McCann *et al.*, 2007). As you have probably gathered by now, the intercultural nature of this book is incompatible with a deficiency view of service user communication. Instead, we have chosen to adopt Hall's (1959) view that culture is analogous to music. Each culture has its own rhythms, patterns and use of time or silences. These musical aspects of communication can be the icing on the linguistic cake (Tannen, 2005), adding colour and flavour to interactions. And just as the decoration on a fancy wedding cake can have an impact that is even more powerful and memorable than the cake itself, the musical elements of communication can carry a far more lasting message than the words themselves.

This is the first of three chapters that focus upon non-verbal communication. All elements are inter-linked, and Table 4.1 illustrates how these are divided up and explored within this book.

Table 4.1: How chapters link within this book: Chapter 4

Chapter 3: Word-based Interpersonal Communication	Chapter 4: Musical Aspects of Communication	Chapter 5: Body Language	Chapter 6: Environmental Aspects of Communication	Chapter 7: Professional Scripts
• The role of words • Inclusive and exclusive communication • Scripting	• **Pitch/Key** • **Vocal qualifiers** • **Volume** • **Pace/Rate/ Timing** • **Silence**	• Proxemics (distance) • Kinesics (movements and gesture) • Haptics (touch) • Facial expression	• Physical environment • Objects • Territoriality • Sensory input as communication	• Putting the chapters together to perform your role

In Chapter 3 you were introduced to the work of Hymes (2005) and the ten components that constitute communication. The musical aspects of speech have particular links with the message form, key, norms of speech, interaction and interpretation. You may find it helpful to refer to this information in Table 3.1 to refresh your memory on this topic before reading further.

Music and Emotions: Family Lens

This exercise is designed to get you thinking about how sensitised you are to listening to musical elements in life in general before we go on to consider musical aspects of speech. Think about how important music is within your life.

? **How often do you listen to music? (e.g. on the radio or other devices)**

? **How intensely do you listen? (e.g. background music, going to concerts, listening in a quiet room with nothing else going on)**

? **Can you identify any musical pieces that you link with a particular emotion? If so,**

? **What pieces of music do you associate with the following emotions:**

- Happiness
- Sadness
- Anger

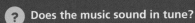

Music and Culture: National Lens

Listen to a piece of music from a culture that is very different to your own. If you are from a Western culture, listen to a piece that is an example of traditional Chinese or Asian music. If you are from an Eastern culture, listen to a piece of English, American or European folk music. As you listen, think about the following:

? **Does the music sound in tune?**

? **Are there predictable patterns to the music, or is everything a bit of a surprise?**

? **How comfortable do you feel?**

? **What emotion do you experience? (e.g. enjoyment, boredom, disquiet)**

Box 4.1: Your music under different cultural lenses

INNATE MUSICALITY

Whether you consider yourself to be an aspiring rock god, classical maestro or as sensitive as a brick to everything musical, you are surrounded by elements of music from the earliest stages of life. One of the first sounds you hear is the rhythm of the maternal heartbeat whilst still in the womb (Ochs, 1993). Music is basic and primordial. When we hear birdsong, with its complex patterns and reciprocal exchanges of notes between different members of the group, we are listening to a form of communication that harks back to the dawn of humanity (Geissmann, 2000). Musicality is evident within our very earliest developmental stages. From the second week of life, babies' cries start to show increasingly complex melody arcs that can be interpreted as communication by attentive care givers (Wermke *et al.*, 2007). We are all pre-programmed to hear and respond to musical elements such as changes in pitch, volume, pace and rhythm. Babies as young as 5 months prefer musical sounds to pure speech and respond with different emotions to different types of musical input (Moog, 1976). They don't understand what they are hearing, but they feel it and respond to it without conscious thought. As the typically developing child matures, this pre-symbolic emotional response to music changes to a response that is in line with cultural norms. As you are exposed to music you learn the type of emotional meaning that your culture attributes to that sound. In Western culture for example, sad music is linked to minor keys, with slow beats, whilst happy music is often in a major key (Cooke, 1959). This requires an understanding of musical symbolism, just as verbal symbolism is needed in order to understand that a word denotes an object. The ability to identify culturally learned emotional responses to musical pieces comes on line around the age of 3 (Kastner *et al.*, 1990; Kratus, 1993). The important points to note here are that an individual can hear musical sounds and feel an emotion without having any understanding of formal language (John'a,

Emotional Message Beats Factual Message

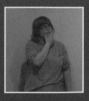

If you doubt the power of the musical aspects of speech, try the following exercise:

Pick a partner to communicate with. It's probably best to warn them in advance that you're trying out a communication exercise, or you may end up getting into trouble!

? **Pay them a compliment e.g. 'you've been a great help to me'.**

? **However, your tone of voice should be sending the opposite message (e.g. you were useless).**

? **Ask them what message they picked up from what you said.**

If you've acted this well, the message that they report will not be positive, despite the way this may look if written down.

If they picked up on the positive message, one or both of you could do with working on your acting!

Box 4.2: The power of music over words

1991; Juslin *et al.*, 2010; Sloboda *et al.*, 2001). This is a common factor that binds all of us as humans respond to music and musical elements of speech, even if the ability to consciously interpret and articulate the emotional response is absent. However, there may also be culturally learned ways of listening out for and hearing musical aspects of speech. This has implications for health and social care settings when staff are interacting with service users who may have difficulty with conscious and symbolic communication. Have a go at the exercises in Box 4.1 to help you understand how your exposure to music links to your emotions.

The innate musical hotwiring means that you continue to be bombarded by musical influences throughout your life (Trevarthen, 1979; Trevarthen, 2000). Rhythm is perceived by the vast majority of people, including those who are deaf (Korduba, 1975), or who have a profound learning disability (Graham, 2004). Even those who have brain damage that prevents them from perceiving music (amusia) are able to hear and respond to musical elements of speech (Ayotte *et al.*, 2002). The universality of the musical elements of speech acts as a double-edged sword. It can help to bridge cultural differences and aid communication in situations where there is not a common language. However, if it is not managed well, it can communicate our true feelings to others without us intending to. The following quotation illustrates how a service user who is used to attending to the musical aspects of speech picked up on the emotions of staff:

They said that they wanted to help me but they sounded cross. They didn't really care. I think they were busy.

Communicate2U quotation 4.1: Service user picking up on staff tone of voice

The message that staff in the quotation wished to convey is unlikely to be the one that the service user picked up. The danger of viewing any service user group in terms of their deficits (for examples see Cain *et al.*, 2007; Eigsti *et al.*,

2011) is that relative strengths that individuals may have can be overlooked. We also run the risk of evaluating communication from a stance of cultural superiority, rather than assuming cultural difference (Jandt, 2007; Labov, 1972). As the quotation above illustrates, this can lead to difficult encounters in health or social care settings since the message that is picked up during the crucial opening moments of an interaction is negative, and time is then wasted in trying to get the interaction on track. To experience this for yourself, have a go at the exercise in Box 4.2, and consider how comfortable you would be in interacting with someone whose words said something positive, but whose tone of voice indicated the opposite.

The sections that follow are designed to help you to understand your own cultural tendencies in relation to the musical aspects of speech, and how these may be used to improve communication encounters with people who find words hard, or don't use words at all.

INTENTIONAL AND UNINTENTIONAL COMMUNICATION

Non-verbal elements of speech usually account for around 67% of the message that is transmitted (Devito, 1997), but for people who struggle to communicate with words, this figure can be over 90% (Bild, 2010). The message that is transmitted non-verbally tends to be emotional, rather than factual (Devito, 1997), and where there is dissonance between these two elements, the emotional message is the one that people believe (Danziger, 1976; Leathers *et al.*, 2008). Musicality trumps words every time because it bypasses our conscious awareness and speaks directly to the primitive part of the brain that is linked to basic survival mechanisms. This does not mean that the musical elements of speech are pure and free from misinterpretation – they too are susceptible to inaccurate interpretation (Danziger, 1976), particularly if people come from different cultural backgrounds. However, basic emotions such as anger, pain and happiness can generally be communicated between people from a wide range of cultures (Berger *et al.*, 1969), provided that the communication partner is open to listening to them. Unfortunately, the word-dominated world of health and social care is not always able to listen to the musical elements of communication

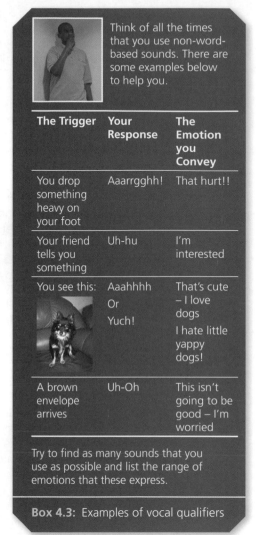

Think of all the times that you use non-word-based sounds. There are some examples below to help you.

The Trigger	Your Response	The Emotion you Convey
You drop something heavy on your foot	Aaarrgghh!	That hurt!!
Your friend tells you something	Uh-hu	I'm interested
You see this:	Aaahhhh Or Yuch!	That's cute – I love dogs I hate little yappy dogs!
A brown envelope arrives	Uh-Oh	This isn't going to be good – I'm worried

Try to find as many sounds that you use as possible and list the range of emotions that these express.

Box 4.3: Examples of vocal qualifiers

that those who find words hard use. This inability to hear communication that is in the form of sounds rather than articulated words can contribute to unnecessary pain and suffering, or even premature and avoidable death if staff overlook basic emotional communication from vulnerable people (Francis, 2013; Mencap, 2006).

Communication does not have to be in the form of words. The vocabulary of our everyday exchanges is littered with **vocal qualifiers** – seemingly nonsense sounds that in fact convey an emotional message (Devito, 1997). Have a go at the exercise in Box 4.3 to identify some of the ones that you use. Communication can also be in the form of silence (an aspect of communication which will be explored in more depth later in this chapter), in a grunt, a howl (Berger *et al.*, 1969) or a random sound that is shared between two people and sent back and forth. This latter form of communication is called **mirroring**, and it can be the starting point for a communication exchange with people who have no formal language. It is commonly seen to occur between adults and young babies. The baby initiates a sound that the adult imitates, and soon there is an extended interaction with the sound being bounced backwards and forwards, being modified and turns being taken. The young baby is not consciously intending to communicate, but communication happens. This form of unintentional communication is therefore generally a part of our family and national culture. It is interesting to note that whilst many qualified staff in health and social care cultural settings appear to struggle to communicate with people with a profound and multiple learning disability (Finlay *et al.*, 2007; Finlay *et al.*, 2008a; Michael *et al.*, 2008), students who had no formal health or social care background were able to communicate well with this client group with less than an hour's training (Zeedyk S. *et al.*, 2009; Zeedyk S. M. *et al.*, 2009). The techniques that they used were based on mirroring as described above and are called intensive interaction. As a teacher at a special school notes, the basic skills required to communicate with people who have no formal language are not based on a lot of technical knowledge, but on instinctive forms of communication.

Intensive interaction's a very particular term for what are very basic skills that every parent of a new-born child does instinctively, do you know what I mean? (Peter – Teacher at a Special School for People with Learning Disability)

Communicate2U quotation 4.2: Peter: the innate basic communication skills we all possess

Mirroring does not only occur with infants or those who work well with vulnerable communicators. It is a part of our everyday repertoire of communication. When we communicate well with someone, we usually unconsciously mirror their tone, pitch, pace, volume and timing. In the process of becoming a professional who is adept at using precise, technical word-based language, it is also important to recognise these seemingly everyday musical communication skills have value in organisational and professional cultures. You need to recognise what musical skills you have, why they are important, and how you can transfer the skills that you use from one cultural setting to another. This will help you to make the emotional (and potentially unintentional) aspects of speech an intentional part of your communication repertoire. This should help you to communicate more effectively with people who don't have intentional speech, such as people with a profound learning disability or late-stage dementia. It will help you to manage the emotional message that you convey to all service users and carers with whom you come into contact to ensure that you do not inadvertently send out the wrong type of information. It may also help you to think about the importance of body language and environmental communication (Chapters 5 and 6) with people who are deaf and therefore unable to pick up on the emotional message that is present in your voice. The sections that follow will look at the musical elements of speech in more depth to support you in this process.

PITCH

Pitch is the equivalent of how far up or down the musical scale the sounds we make are: high pitched and the notes are up high on the scale, or even above the lines; low pitched and the notes are lower down.

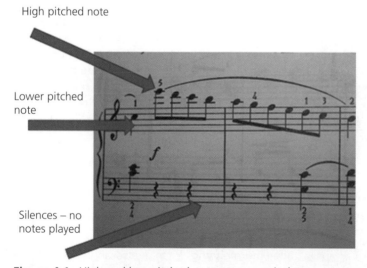

Figure 4.1: High and low pitched notes on a musical score

As a general communication principle, it is important to remember that as people get older, they find it harder to hear notes at the extreme ends of the scale. The loss of ability to discriminate pitch also makes it harder to filter out background noises (Moore, 2008; Oxenham, 2008) making it important to try to

Pitch and Key

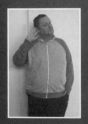

Listen to the audio clip on the website. You will hear the same words spoken several times, but in different ways. After each example, write down what message and emotion you think is actually being conveyed.

Find a small group of willing people and explain that you are going to say the same words to them in different ways. You will read the words in the table below, stressing the ones written in bold. After each phrase, you want them to say what kind of message was being conveyed. See if it matches the ideas we have come with at Communicate2U.

You can go now	You can go (but the others can't), I'm going to do something extra with you
You **can** go now	You can go now (but you weren't allowed to before) I'm a bit annoyed that you're asking.
You can **go** now	I'm fed up with you being here
You can go **now**	Just hurry up and go! Get lost!

Members of Communicate2U have sometimes not understood that an appointment has ended. They have had these words said in very unfriendly ways that have upset them. They would like you to practise saying them in ways that won't upset others.

Have a go at playing around with different pitches and find the ones that make this phrase sound as friendly as possible.

Box 4.4: Pitch, key and sounding friendly to vulnerable service users

communicate in quiet environments. Facing the person who has the hearing difficulty, and talking at a normal pace can make it easier for them to lip read. The visual strategies that were outlined at the end of Chapter 3, such as using pictures alongside words, can also help to give additional information to support communication. However, pitch also plays a much more subtle role in communication. Pitch plays its part in accentuating, complementing, controlling and regulating the overall message that is sent (Devito, 1997). The way that it does this is determined by cultural rules (Jandt, 2007).

Some cultures make more overt use of pitch to communicate than others. For example, Mandarin makes extensive use of pitch changes within speech (Bent *et al.*, 2006) as do some Indian languages (Gumperz, 1978) and Arabic (Jandt, 2007). The same sound can mean something entirely different if the pitch changes. For example, the word 'tang' in Chinese means 'soup' if the note stays high, but 'sugar' if the note goes higher as you say it (a friendly note of caution: I want to kiss you/I want to tell you, also use exactly the same sounds!). Whilst English speakers may not appear to make such extensive use of pitch to communicate, pitch plays a vital role in conveying meaning and marking out different points in a conversation. As you saw at the end of Chapter 3, the English language has many words that have multiple meanings (**polysemy**), and there tends to be quite a relaxed approach to word order (Chomsky, 1965). Therefore, changes in pitch offer important cues as to meaning. This is inextricably linked to the key of the communication exchange – in other words, the emotional meaning that is conveyed. The exercise in Box 4.4 illustrates this point. Each time an important word is conveyed, the pitch is changed subtly to alter the meaning. Pitch is also an important cue in terms of conveying changes in the stages of an interaction. In English, rising pitch at the end of a phrase indicates a question, cuing the speech partner to respond, whilst falling pitch indicates the end of a phrase, which may invite the speech partner to take their turn to introduce a new point (Devito, 1997). English speakers, however, tend to be relatively poor at picking up pitch cues in comparison to cultures in which pitch plays a more prominent role. When different cultural groups meet, there can be culture clashes. Gumperz (1978) describes a scene in an English café in which a Pakistani speaker of English asks customers if they want gravy with their meal. The server does so with a falling inflection at the end of the word (indicating a statement), rather than the rising inflection that the English customers are accustomed to associating with a question (Gravy?). Customers judged the servers to be surly and incompetent, and responded accordingly. The servers in return felt that they were being discriminated against. In this case, differences in cultural expectations associated with pitch led to some serious miscommunication that adversely affected employee relationships, and required management intervention. This type of miscommunication can occur in many different types of intercultural exchanges.

Within health and social care settings, similar intercultural misunderstandings can occur when staff and vulnerable communicators meet. People who find verbal communication difficult may not always follow pitch cues to take their turn in ways that staff are expecting. People with a learning disability, for example, may have a relatively limited range of pitch, and come across as monotonous to other listeners. They may also not pick up the pitch cue that indicates that a speaker is yielding the floor to another speaker and so may jump into the conversation before staff expect them to (Brumback et al., 1983). This may result in them being labelled as rude, or people with whom it is difficult to communicate. Within their family cultural environments, service users and supporters may well have developed more exaggerated pitch cues to indicate a change in speaker. Health and social care staff may not have developed the necessary sensitivity to pick up and mirror this linguistic form. Service users and carers who are expecting staff to support the person with the learning disability to engage in the conversation may be labelled as people who have difficulty in listening (Devito, 1997). The end result is the same as that outlined in Gumperz's example – both parties are unhappy, and both feel the other is to blame.

PACE, TIMING AND SILENCES WITHIN CONVERSATIONAL STAGES

Health and social care literature into best communication practice recognises the need to allow more time for interactions with people with additional needs, such as those who are deaf (Fellinger et al., 2012), have dementia (de Vries, 2013; Moyle et al., 2008) or a learning disability (Blair, 2011). This is generally framed in terms of needing more overall time to meet the expected outcomes for an intervention. However, what is less well explored are the hidden cultural rules that govern the pace, timing and silences of interactions.

Each cultural group has its own natural patterns for communication, and these occur at a culturally determined pace, in a culturally determined order. For example, in Western cultures, conversations generally occur as shown in Figure 4.2:

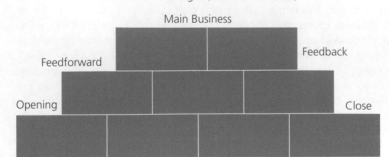

Conversational Stages (after Devito 1997)

Figure 4.2: The stages of conversation in Western culture

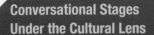

Conversational Stages Under the Cultural Lens

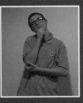

At the end of Chapter 1 you were asked to identify your cultural mixing desk. If you haven't done so, go to Figure 1.14 and do that now.

Pick two cultural groups to which you belong that have very different cultural profiles.

For each of them have a think about the following:

? How fast do members of that group tend to talk when they are together?

? Which members of the group tend to open up conversations? (for example, is this shared, or does someone tend to lead?)

? Who tends to control the flow and speed of interactions?

? Does every group member get an equal share of the interaction time?

The more dominant speakers are like the conductor of the orchestra: they tend to control the conversational score and who gets to play.

Box 4.5: Controlling the musical score within interactions

However, within this simple diagram there is a wealth of hidden cultural norms. Openings are associated with greetings, and these are ritualised and patterned (Goffman, 1967). During the feedforward stage, someone will introduce the idea that is to be discussed – that may be in a very formal way (for example, when the agenda of a business meeting is read out), or in an informal way ('let's decide where to go for lunch'). The main business will then usually consist of interaction partners taking turns to contribute to the conversation as ideas are exchanged back and forth (Devito, 1997). Ideas will be clarified (feedback), and the exchange will be brought to a close with a formalised parting (e.g. 'see you next time'). This will be examined in more depth in chapter seven where we look at changing the script in health and social care interactions to include vulnerable communicators. In successful exchanges the whole process often takes place without conscious effort because there is an unconscious rhythm to the interaction. Rhythm is bound up with pace, timing and silences, and when it goes wrong, the results can be as grating as a poorly matched orchestra desperately trying to follow a difficult score. Before exploring pace and timing in more depth, we will examine the underpinning glue that holds those elements together – silence.

Silence

For something that is essentially nothing, silence is incredibly powerful. Within music, silences can convey an emotional message. The main theme in Beethoven's 5th Symphony has slight pauses between the main musical message (da da da ... daaah ... check it out online – this does not work in words!). Without the pause, the dramatic moment would not have been as effective. The pattern within this rhythm can also be represented as dot, dot, dot, dash – the letter V in Morse code, a symbolism that had immense importance in the UK during the second world war as it represented victory (Cossins, 2012). John Cage goes as far as to write an entire piece based on 273 seconds of silence (–273°C being the number that is used to denote absolute zero – the point at which everything stops). The next time that you listen to music, listen out for the pauses, the slight silences, and reflect on whether the piece would be as effective if they were absent. Silences convey a large amount of emotional weight in interpersonal exchanges too. Silence can be seen as positive (e.g. contemplative), negative (e.g. sulking) and can be an important factor in the deeper aspects of cultural life such as rituals. During conversation, silences can denote the way in which information is parcelled up, or emphasise a key point. Longer silences can also indicate that it is time to change the speaker – in other words, they serve to let the other person know that it is now their turn to talk (Devito, 1997). However, many people are uncomfortable with silences within conversations, and seek to fill the void with words to make themselves feel better. Norms for uncomfortable silence vary widely between cultures (Scollon et al., 2012), but after around 4 seconds of pause, a Western communicator will often leap in. For a communication partner who needs time to process a comment or question, this is inadequate thinking time. In health and social care exchanges where silence occurs, staff may assume that this means that the person cannot communicate at all and turn to another person in the room to give information instead (e.g. a carer). They may also turn to the relative or carer as this person is more likely to communicate at a pace with which staff are comfortable. The vulnerable communicator can get crowded out of the exchange. They, or the person that supports them may be very aware of this happening, and they can develop an awareness of the importance of silence that may be hidden to more vocal communicators. The quotation below illustrates how the academic author of this book (Annette) learned about the importance of silence from a non-academic author from Communicate2U who has a learning disability (Jill). Annette and Jill are discussing how Jill communicates with a classmate who has very little formal language:

Jill:	*He can still do acting ... if a child can't really, like, talk a bit. They know what they can do. They can just have their ... movements, or silence or anything.*
Annette:	*Silence, now, that's an interesting one, isn't it? Because we always think about the words, but we don't think about the silence so much ... That's an interesting point, though. I'd never thought of it like that before. I'm learning a lot.*
Jill:	*Good.*

Communicate2U quotation 4.3: Jill teaches Annette about the importance of silence

How Comfortable are You with Conversational Silence?

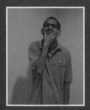 Before you start this exercise, get a feel for time by looking at your watch and finding a word that takes you 1 second to say in your head. ('Mississippi' can be quite a useful word for this!)

Next time you go out with a group of friends, count silently to 5 before responding to statements or questions that come up in the conversation.

? Note how much of the conversation you actually get to take part in.

? What happens when you don't respond immediately? How do you feel? How do those around you react?

? Reflect on how long you normally wait for a response from others before you make another comment or ask another question.

? What impact do you think these skills will have on your work with vulnerable communicators?

When you ask vulnerable service users a question you can do the following:

? Look and see how long people who know them well wait for a reply. Wait a similar length of time.

? Don't ask another question unless their body language clearly suggests they have lost interest in you.

Match the pace of the vulnerable person.

Box 4.6: Your tolerance for silence

In cultures where words dominate, the finer nuances of silences may not always be recognised. Health and social care staff may be taught to consciously use silence as a tool for specific types of interactions such as counselling (Back *et al.*, 2009; Kurtz *et al.*, 2005) but may forget to apply that to general interactions. The small silences may only add up to a short extra period of time for an overall interaction, but they can have a strong positive effect if used well. Even with non-vulnerable people, changing a waiting silence from a norm of 1 second to 3 seconds or more can help to reduce the risk of less confident communicators being excluded from exchanges (Rowe, 1986). For those who are vulnerable and at real risk of not being included at all, allowing a longer silence for a response may give people the opportunity for inclusion in decisions that are made about their personal health and well-being that they may otherwise have missed.

In health and social care settings, allowing more time for the interaction as a whole will be ineffective unless the staff member knows their pace, can feel the natural pace of the communication partner and adapt to their speed. To do this, they must first know their own cultural norms. Have a go at the exercise in Box 4.6 to help you become familiar with your tolerance for silence and how this will link to your role as a professional who wishes to communicate well. Having explored silence, we will now explore how much noise we actually make when we fill the silent void with our voices.

Volume

Volume helps to communicate meaning (Devito, 1997). Increasing volume slightly to stress a particular word can alter the whole meaning of a sentence as you discovered in Box 4.1. However, the cultural rules that govern the use of volume are complex. Emphasis can be achieved through altering volume up or down, and the same emotion may be indicated by volumes at opposite ends of the spectrum. For example, anger may be more traditionally associated with loud voices, but may equally be expressed through a lowered volume – a quietly controlled and tightly spoken phrase that conveys menace. Volume can be a matter of personal style. If you listen to a group of people talking, you will notice too that some people appear to naturally speak more quietly, whilst others seem to have their volume control permanently set to maximum. However, there may also be a cultural dimension to the volume at which an interaction occurs. Some cultures may have a specific preference for a set volume for communication. Looking through the organisational and professional lens, the quietly spoken murmurs within a cloister, and the shouting of an army sergeant major who is training new recruits are examples

How Loud Are You?

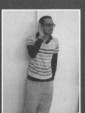 To get your musical ear tuned in, observe a couple of different groups of people interacting in the same setting (for example a pub, or café). Think about the following:

- **?** **Is everybody talking at the same volume?**
- **?** **Does the volume of the group as a whole remain constant, or does it change?**
- **?** **Who are the louder members of the group, and how much of the conversation do they seem to dominate?**

? **Who are the quieter members, and how much of the conversation do they seem to dominate?**

Now start to become aware as to how loud you generally are in the following cultural settings:

- Close family
- Friendship group(s)
- Hobby group(s)
- Work settings

Having thought about your own volume levels, think about the following questions:

- **?** **If your volume levels differ in different groups – why is this?**
- **?** **If they don't – why not?**
- **?** **How aware are you as to the appropriateness of your volume levels in different settings?**

Organisational and Professional Lens

Now think about working with service users who may use or need a different volume to you in the work setting.

- **?** **If you were with a service user and were talking too softly – how would you know?**
- **?** **If you were talking too loudly – how would you know?**
- **?** **Using an intercultural approach, how would you work with a service user who you felt was communicating too loudly for the setting?**

Box 4.7: How loud are you in different cultural settings?

from both ends of the spectrum. Looking through the family lens, some families may be naturally loud and generally get on well, whilst in other families, shouting may be associated with domestic violence (Koolhof et al., 2013). Volume is therefore tricky when considered from an intercultural perspective, but it is extremely important to consider the impact of two different cultural styles meeting.

Health and social care staff will often work in a range of different physical environments, some of which may be quiet, some noisy. Against a background of ambient noise, staff may naturally raise their voice to compensate. For service users from a family culture in which a raised voice is a precursor to conflict, this may cause feelings of discomfort, and staff may be seen as aggressive or threatening. Conversely, service users who have difficulty in interpreting social norms (such as people with a learning disability or dementia) may not recognise that they are expected to lower their voice in a hospital or social care group setting. Staff may view such loud individuals as being rude or disrespectful to other service users. In both cases, viewing the behaviour of the other communicator without considering whether this is a clash of cultural communication styles can lead to negative impressions of the interaction. Volume will be one element of musical communication that contributes to the whole emotional message being conveyed. In extreme cases it may be possible to isolate this as a factor, but it may well end up being a general part of the overall impression of a person's musical style of communication. Honing your listening skills by using the exercises in this chapter should help you to become more aware of your own use of volume and how you may vary this in the different cultural groups to which you belong.

Pace and Timing

People from the same cultural group often share a linguistic style and pace. For example, members of the New York Jewish community have a tendency to speak at a rapid pace, finishing one another's sentences as they leap ahead and guess where the conversation is going. This works really well when all members of the interaction are from that background, but strangers may find themselves getting crowded out of the conversation, unable to get a word in edgeways. The overlapping fast speech style can be interpreted as aggressive and dehumanising by those who are more familiar with a slower pace (Tannen, 2005). The problem tends to be intensified because when people with different cultural paces clash, they tend to intensify their natural behaviour. Fast speakers leave too short a pause for the slower speaker to respond. They are uncomfortable with the longer than usual silence, so leap in to fill it. The slower speaker gets less and less time to respond, so becomes increasingly hesitant (Andelson, 2002).

In Chapter 3 we explored the outcomes that each communication partner may have in relation to an interaction. Health and social care staff are often faced with organisational drivers that require them to complete tasks quickly and efficiently. Time is precious, a commodity not to be wasted. Staff need to take time to be caring and compassionate. Time is expected to do a lot of different things. Given these competing drivers, it is perhaps no wonder that a service user's view of time and what is adequate for an exchange may be very different to a staff view. However, taking an additional few seconds to allow a service user to respond, and becoming familiar with an uncomfortable feeling whilst waiting for this to occur can actually be a valuable investment in time. It can help to make an encounter more humanising, and avoid the kind of experiences that Trudy and Walter outline:

I think when people do meet Walter, they probably assume he doesn't understand as much as he does. So he tends ... after the initial hello, I think, possibly, he can sort of be left out a little bit. (Trudy)

Communicate2U quotation 4.4: Walter being excluded from interactions

When Trudy communicates with Walter at home, she is familiar with how long it takes him to respond, and gives him the time he needs to think and get involved in the interaction. When they are in support meetings, hospital meetings or with a group of friends, people often remember to give Walter an initial greeting at the opening stage of the exchange but then the pace of conversation leaves him behind for all of the main business stage of the interaction. He is only thought of again when it gets to the closing stage when he receives his formal 'goodbye'. Walter and Trudy both notice this because it clashes with their usual style of communicating with each other. These types of experiences can heighten service user and carer sensitivity towards paces, silences and inclusion in a way that people who are confident with using words may not experience.

HEARING THE MUSICAL EMOTIONAL MESSAGE

Developing an ear for hearing the emotional message that is conveyed through the musical aspects of speech will take time. It does not come naturally to many Western listeners (Gumperz, 1978), and there is a limit as to how much of this can be conveyed in text. Giving a non-swimmer who has just fallen in the water a book to read on how to swim is not going to be effective (or welcome!). Just as a swimmer learns competence in the water, you will need to develop your cultural ear for the musical aspects of speech by listening. There is no lack of material to work with – we are surrounded by access to TV, internet and other media that give us insights into other cultures. This can often make it easier to spot obvious differences. You can start by becoming aware as to how your own pitch, timing and silences change in different situations. For example, when you are with friends discussing an exciting new piece of news, do you talk in faster and higher pitched voices? If there is some unwelcome, sad news to discuss, does the pitch become lower and the speed of talking slower? The exercises in Box 4.5 are designed to help you develop these skills in different cultural groups and settings.

Hearing the Musical Message through Cultural Lenses

National and Linguistic Lenses

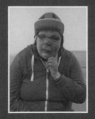

Find some clips of people from different national or language groups interacting. Try to use clips of languages with which you are unfamiliar (Italian, German and Mandarin are good contrasting language styles). As you hear the sounds wash over you listen out for the following:

? **How much variety in pitch is there?**

? **What cues do people give each other to change speaker (e.g. falling pitch, a pause)?**

? **How quickly do people speak?**

? **How long are the pauses between speakers?**

Family, Organisational and Professionals Lenses

Now, use the questions above to become aware of your own styles in the following settings:

? **At home**

? **At a work meeting with other professionals**

? **At a work meeting with service users or carers who find words hard**

Box 4.8: Musical messages through different cultural lenses

In this book we are arguing that all vulnerable communicators who are capable of making sounds can communicate an emotional message to people who are good at listening out for it. For people who do not have intentional communication, non-word-based sounds (and body language) may be one of their primary forms of expressing themselves to the outside world. That does not mean to say that interpreting and understanding this message is an easy process. We may think we understand what a sound means, but that interpretation may be based on a hidden cultural assumption that does not translate to other cultures. Non-word-based sounds can become a part of the general culture without people being aware of it (Berger *et al.*, 1969). For example, a growl may generally be interpreted by the main cultural group to mean anger. However, for a communicator who has a limited repertoire of sounds and no intentional communication, a growl may be their natural way of expressing pleasure. This type of communicator is reliant upon those that know them well to understand their unique communicative style, and even then there may be discrepancies in interpretation (Johnson *et al.*, 2010). However, someone who is well attuned to the sounds a vulnerable communicator makes is generally in a much stronger position to interpret that emotional communication effectively. Unfortunately, staff in health and social care settings are not always willing to acknowledge that expertise. Carers who have heard a person in pain and insisted that their relative is in distress have been ignored, as staff have assumed that the sounds are meaningless. There has been an assumption that professional expertise is more accurate than the lived experience of vulnerable communicators and their relatives or carers. This stance of cultural superiority has in extreme cases led to the avoidable death of vulnerable people (Francis, 2013; Mencap, 2006). Whilst not identified specifically as cultural translation tools, there are some communication support systems that have been developed to help the different cultural worlds understand each other more effectively. Communication passports and the Disability Distress

Assessment Tool (DisDAT) (Regnard *et al.*, 2007), for example, allow carers to explain how a vulnerable communicator communicates non-verbally. The structured format of such tools not only provides a translation when carers are absent, but the formalised nature of the process may make it more acceptable to health and social care staff who are accustomed to technical learning. However, staff will only use the tools if they are prepared to hear sounds and silences as communication, which is not always the case (Finlay *et al.*, 2007; Windley *et al.*, 2010). Staff can fall into the trap of only seeing people who use words and can communicate using factual information as communicating beings, ignoring those who use sounds to send an emotional message.

There is a second type of trap that staff may fall into if they fail to see the musical aspects of speech. They may overlook situations in which the carer or relative is not attentive to these elements of communication with the vulnerable communicator. Good communication is characterised by mirroring and synchronous patterns between the communication partners. When this is absent it can be a sign of relationship breakdown or a warning to be on the alert for issues of neglect or abuse (Cooney *et al.*, 2006). If vulnerable communicators cannot be understood by those people that spend the majority of the time with them, then their needs are unlikely to be fully met, and they will have no way of expressing this to the outside world. If health and social care staff rely upon the reports of the relative or carer without assessing how they interact with the vulnerable communicator, they will not have assessed the situation fully. However, even if staff do assess the quality of communication and note a lack of synchronicity, that does not always indicate a poor relationship. As the quotation below illustrates, in rare cases some people have styles of communication in which it is extremely difficult to discern any type of pattern. Dean describes some of his pupils with profound learning disability with whom he struggles to communicate:

I mean, the really challenging ones are the ones that you think, gosh, I really don't know what, you know, makes you tick, ... it can be really, really hard to know, you know, what motivates them, what things they like doing, because you might think, oh, you like X, Y, and Z, but then the next day, they're completely uninterested in that. I mean, that's only a small proportion. (Dean – Teacher)

Communicate2U quotation 4.5: Dean trying to understand communication with people who have patterns of communication that are hard to see

The difference between a lack of interest and a lack of synchronicity in communication styles is clearly shown here. Dean is clearly trying to find out how to communicate with his students who have no formal speech. He is alert to their non-verbal communication – their sounds and movements – and he tries hard to find a link between these and the activities that the students are undertaking. The lack of a pattern frustrates him as it thwarts his ability to communicate and respond appropriately. Asking a carer or relative what the sounds that a person makes mean, or how long you should wait for a response may give health and social care staff a valuable insight into how that individual is viewed. If the relative or carer sees them as a communicating being and is trying hard to understand the musical aspects of speech as communication, they are indicating that they care. If they are dismissive of the sounds as having any communicative function or cannot see this themselves, they are condemning the person to an extremely isolated existence at best.

CHAPTER SUMMARY: AIMING FOR INTERACTIVE HARMONY

Looking at all the words that have been written about the musical aspects of speech, it may be tempting to view this as a difficult concept that is hard to apply to people who communicate in ways that are different to your own. However, don't forget that words are a poor way to convey music. Just as music has to be rehearsed and performed to be appreciated, the best way to improve your performance in becoming an effective intercultural musical performer is to listen and practise. First, listen to yourself and your different styles in different cultural settings. Become aware that you have these musical skills, and start to appreciate them for what they are: a key to unlocking communication with people who are often left out of interactions in health and social care settings completely: people with severe learning disability, late stage dementia or complex neurological or mental health needs. Listen to their style, their pace, sounds and rhythm, and then try to match it. Viewing the person with these additional skills as an expert in their own cultural communication style may eventually pay dividends. You may find that there are people out there whose affinity for the musical aspects of speech outstrips your own ability (for example, people with a form of learning disability called Williams Syndrome (Mackenzie, 2007; Martens et al., 2011)). You will learn to hear a much greater variety of emotional communication, and have the satisfaction of knowing that even if you are not completely sure you have understood the whole message, you have heard more of it than you would have done previously. Mirroring the musical style of the vulnerable communicator will be appreciated by supportive family and carers who value that aspect of communication themselves. It may make you more alert to situations in which very vulnerable people are living with carers who do not wish to, or are not able to, listen to their emotional needs. Synchronicity and harmony of style makes communication a much more satisfying experience for all parties concerned, and is well worth the extra effort. This theme will continue in the next chapter when we consider the non-verbal aspects of communication that are conveyed not through sound, but through observing the body as it communicates.

Easy Read Chapter Summary

 Grrrrrrrrrrrrrrrrrrrrrrr!	How you say words is often more important than the words themselves
	Speech uses silences, different sounds and volumes – just like music
	The musical parts of speech show our emotions
	Everybody uses this kind of communication – even people who can't speak using words
	Silence can be really important as well as sounds

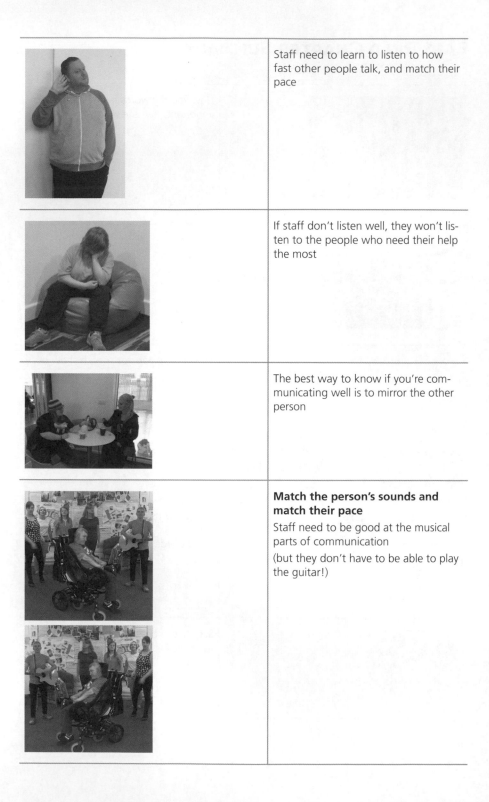

	Staff need to learn to listen to how fast other people talk, and match their pace
	If staff don't listen well, they won't listen to the people who need their help the most
	The best way to know if you're communicating well is to mirror the other person
	Match the person's sounds and match their pace Staff need to be good at the musical parts of communication (but they don't have to be able to play the guitar!)

CHAPTER

5

BODY LANGUAGE

Aims

By the end of this chapter you will be able to:

➡ Identify how we use our bodies to communicate

➡ Explain why body language is an important part of the overall message

➡ Reflect upon how you use your own body to communicate in different cultural settings

➡ Critically evaluate the impact of your body language in interactions with service users

INTRODUCTION

In Chapter 4 you were introduced to the interlinking non-verbal constituent components of communication. Table 5.1 is a repeat of Table 4.1 to remind you that whilst we consider the elements separately, in reality these usually occur simultaneously. However, the degree to which each of the aspects is attended to may vary widely, particularly if people have sensory impairment. For example, for people with hearing loss, body language may carry a larger portion of the non-verbal message, whilst for those who are blind or partially sighted the musical aspects of speech and haptics (touch) will carry more of the message. The degree to which people have sensory loss varies widely, and the strategies that people adopt to facilitate communication are linked not only to how much sensory input is available, but also at what life stage the loss occurred (Barnett, 2002a; Bau, 1999). People who have sensory impairment will have developed their own cultural way of communicating, whether within family groupings or wider communities (Barnett, 2002b; Bau, 1999). Health and social care staff who have limited experience of service users with alternative communication strategies may be worried about how to communicate with service users who have sensory impairment (Bryan et al., 2002). Whilst there may be many situations in which it is necessary to seek expert advice from specialists such as speech and language therapists, sign language translators or visual impairment organisations, there will be many more situations in which that support is not immediately

Family Cultural Lens

Scene 1

Imagine that you've organised a family gathering in an unfamiliar village hall and are in the middle of giving a small speech. The lights suddenly go out and you realise that you need to get people outside. It's very dark, and there are some family members who you know may be vulnerable.

 What communication strategies could you use to keep people calm and get people out of the building?

Scene 2

Imagine that you are at a train station and are saying goodbye to a member of your family. There are a lot of trains and people, and the noise is incredible – you've given up trying to talk. As the train arrives you suddenly realise that a piece of luggage is missing.

 What strategies do you use to communicate this knowledge to the person who is about to board the train?

Box 5.1: Communicating in different ways in different settings

available, and you need to communicate with the person in front of you. Considering communication from an intercultural context should help you to recognise your existing communication skills and to apply them in these types of situations. Before we move on to explore skills associated with body language in more depth, have a go at the exercises in Box 5.1 to identify some of your existing competencies. Also use Table 5.1 to remind yourself of the interlinked nature of all the components of communication that are discussed within this book, and where body language is situated.

To help you see the ease with which you naturally link different aspects of communication, let's review the exercises you did in Box 5.1. In Scene 1 you will have probably used many of the musical aspects of speech identified in Chapter 4 to control the situation. You may have raised the volume of your voice to get people's attention, but then consciously slowed your speech down to enable people to have time to attend to your instructions. You will have given enough time for people to respond to any questions that you posed, and listened out for silences that indicated people who may have been too scared to respond (the most vulnerable people in the room). You may have tried to bring the pitch of your voice down from a high level (that indicated stress) to a lower one (that indicated calm) so that your overall key was one of confident control. If you didn't think of these things,

Table 5.1: How chapters link within this book: Chapter 5

Chapter 3: Word-Based Interpersonal Communication	Chapter 4: Musical Aspects of Communication	**Chapter 5: Body Language**	Chapter 6: Environmental Aspects of Communication	Chapter 7: Professional Scripts
• The role of words • Inclusive and exclusive communication • Scripting	• Pitch/Key • Vocal qualifiers • Volume • Pace/Rate/Timing • Silence	• **Proxemics (distance)** • **Kinesics (movements and gesture)** • **Haptics (touch)** • **Facial expression**	• Physical environment • Objects • Territoriality • Sensory input as communication	• Putting the chapters together to perform your role

then it may be worth revising Chapter 4! In this chapter we'll explore some of the things that you may have instinctively done in Scene 2. This may have included tapping the person on the shoulder to get their attention, pointing to other pieces of luggage, miming the size or shape of the missing piece, and using a gesture such as spreading the hands wide to indicate that you don't know its whereabouts. We will examine the way in which you use your body to communicate non-verbally and bring these skills to conscious awareness. This will enable you to use them more effectively, not only with people who are vulnerable because of sensory impairment, but with those who are vulnerable because they find using words hard or impossible.

FACIAL EXPRESSION OF EMOTION

In Chapter 4 it was argued that some aspects of musical communication occur at a pre-conscious level and are therefore picked up as an emotional message by everyone, regardless of the stage of cognitive development someone is operating at, or the culture to which they belong. Some facial expressions also fit into this category, and whilst strictly speaking facial expression should come under the heading of kinesics, it has its own section here to allow us to explore the implications of this innate form of communication.

Of all of our body parts, our face has the greatest capacity to communicate (Knapp *et al.*, 2013). It is capable of some 10,000 expressions, of which around a third express an emotion. However, the decoding of facial emotional expression is often a complex and imprecise skill, with a few notable exceptions (Ekman *et al.*, 2013). It was Charles Darwin who first hypothesised that some emotions must be common to all species that share a common ancestry (Darwin *et al.*, 2009; 1859). For example, the facial expression that is associated with a feeling of anger has many similarities with the ways in which other animals express hostility (for example, a dog baring its teeth) (Izard, 1994). Research into people from widely differing national and ethnic cultural backgrounds strongly suggests that the following basic emotions look the same on the faces of all people, regardless of their culture (Neuliep, 2009).

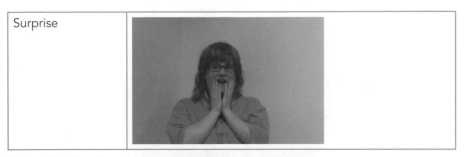

| Surprise | |

Figure 5.1: Emotions that are recognised across cultures

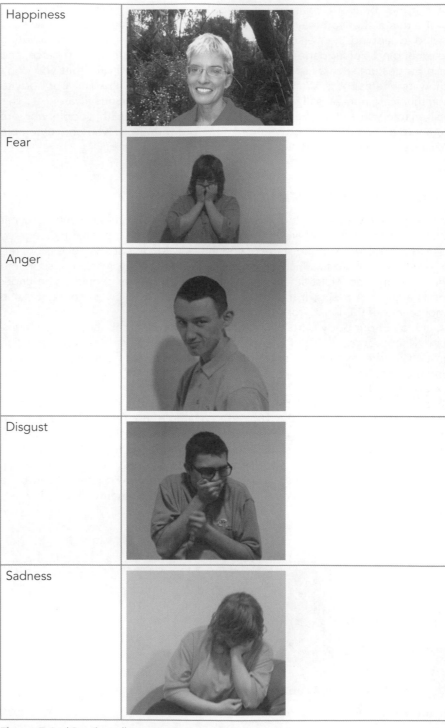

Figure 5.1: (*Continued*)

However, cultures may differ in the degree to which it is acceptable for emotions to be expressed, and the degree to which they recognise these emotions on the faces of others. For example, in cultures which tend to try to avoid uncertainty and have social institutions in place to address this, recognition of fear tends to be less well developed (Matsumoto, 1989). It has already been argued in this book that health and social care settings have a tendency towards high uncertainly avoidance, and there is evidence that some institutions have a poor history of recognising or acting upon the basic emotional communication of some of the most vulnerable service users (Finlay et al., 2007; Mencap, 2013; Mencap, 2006). The exercise in Box 5.2 is designed to get you thinking creatively about what facial expressions and body language may be communicating to you. Try to think of as many possible explanations for each look as you can. Then consider generally how comfortable you are with dealing with emotional expression. If you find this uncomfortable you are more likely to revert to your cultural norm of avoidance when faced with service users. For people who only have emotional communication, you then exclude them entirely from an interaction. Developing a degree of comfort with seeing and responding to emotional communication is a vital skill if you are to avoid excluding vulnerable people from interactions.

When people find it difficult to understand words, they may be particularly sensitised to look for non-verbal clues, such as facial expression, as Quotation 5.1 illustrates. Josie has a mild learning disability. When you first speak to her this isn't noticeable as she has a range of verbal strategies (such as the vocal qualifier 'uh hu' that was highlighted in Chapter 4) that she uses to mask her lack of understanding. She had struggled in a mainstream school before being moved to a special school. She mentioned that she was good at picking up on what emotion people were conveying by looking at their faces:

Annette: So, you're good at picking up people's facial expressions, do you think?

Josie: Oh, yes.

Annette: Yes? What's made you so good at doing that?

Josie: I don't know. I think being at my old school like because I used to like be really paranoid about what people would say and stuff and I used to like look at their face and go, oh, they're saying something good or they're saying something bad or ... and they don't understand what I'm doing. It's just like that.

Communicate2U quotation 5.1: Josie explains why she is good at picking up on facial expressions

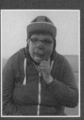

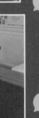
Josie was particularly sensitive about picking up on facial expression. She used this to judge how people were reacting to her as she knew that she sometimes misunderstood things, and this gave her an early indication that this had occurred. This type of strategy may work well when the emotions concerned are the basic ones listed above, but other emotions can be much more difficult for us all to distinguish (Ekman *et al.*, 2013). Some service users may have particular difficulties in distinguishing between more subtle facial expressions because of a whole range of conditions such as autistic spectrum disorder (Adolphs *et al.*, 2001; Eigsti *et al.*, 2011), learning disability (Eigsti *et al.*, 2011; Ozbič *et al.*, 2010), particular forms of dementia (Keane *et al.*, 2002), Parkinson's disease (Sprengelmeyer *et al.*, 2003) or schizophrenia (Edwards *et al.*, 2002) to name but a few. These types of issues mean that many communicatively vulnerable service users will have had previous negative experiences when interacting with strangers (Hall, 2004; Snyder, 2012; Sweeting *et al.*, 2001). They will have failed to pick up on cues that indicate that they needed to alter their interaction style, or may have misinterpreted the emotions of others, leading to an inappropriate reaction. When this occurs the others may well have responded by laughing, or by becoming unfriendly. This may lead to a tendency to view the world as being more hostile than those who have not had this type of experience (Embregts *et al.*, 2009). Have a look at the list of emotions you made in Box 5.2 and note how many emotions can be associated with just one expression.

The range of ways of interpreting facial expression can create problems in health and social care settings. For example, if staff are a little preoccupied, service users may interpret this as being annoyed or uninterested. Either of these interpretations starts the interaction off on a poor footing. Learning to convey a clear basic emotion that is appropriate to the situation is an essential component of the professional script, and one that will be explored in more depth in chapter seven. For now, practise the exercises in Box 5.3 so that you become familiar not only with your own basic facial expressions, but how these are interpreted by others.

There is another issue related to facial recognition of emotions that may create difficulties for staff. Health and social care staff who are used to looking for emotional communication in the faces of service users may experience some discomfort when the cues that they are expecting fail to appear. This occurs in a whole range of conditions in addition to the ones listed above, for example when there is limited mobility in the face because of neurological impairment or scarring (Chambers, 2003), or because the expressions used by a person to express emotion are unique to them. A lack of expected expression can throw us as it contradicts the cultural norms that we are accustomed to (Hymes, 2005). However, an excess of expression can also be disconcerting. We learn to regulate our facial expression of emotion in accordance with cultural norms (Neuliep, 2009). These norms have been shown to exist at a national and ethnic level of culture (Jandt, 2007), but as the exercise in Box 5.4 illustrates, they may also exist at different levels in other cultural groupings. When faced with people who may not control their expression of emotion in ways that we expect (such as some people with a learning disability, mental health support need or dementia) you may feel overwhelmed. In such cases, the service user will have developed their own cultural way of communicating with those that know them well. You will need to learn this code from the service user or family and carers. However, in order to do this, you need to be open to working with a range of unfamiliar communication styles. A failure to do this can lead to the type of culture clashes that can lead to service users being denied equitable access to services because staff are ill-equipped to deal with basic emotional communication (Leucht *et al.*, 2007; Mencap, 2013; Mencap, 2006). A tool such as the Disability Distress Assessment Tool (DisDAT) (Regnard *et al.*, 2007) or communication passports can be useful if the service user lacks words. Where the service user can speak, however, you will need to learn to look for a variety of clues that indicate what emotional message is being conveyed, and to acknowledge your own levels of comfort when faced with a degree of emotional expression which is outside of your cultural norms (use the exercises in Box 5.4 to help you to do this). In order to do that, you will need to get close enough to communicate. This leads us to our next element of body language communication that we will consider: the distance between you and your communication partner.

Now, be brave and either find a friend or a mirror.

Try out the following facial expressions and get feedback (from your own reflections – literally and figuratively! – or your friend).

? **Bored**

? **Thinking hard**

? **Tired**

It's likely that all of these expressions look very similar to a vulnerable service user.

Now try looking interested. Practise this hard because you need to look this every time you meet with service users and carers. If your emotional expression is not clearly one of interest and concern, you are likely to be judged negatively.

Remember: when you assess service users, you are being assessed by them.

Box 5.3: The importance of looking interested

How comfortable are you with emotional displays: under the cultural lens

Family Lens

For each of the four emotions shown below (anger, happiness, sadness, fear), think of an occasion where you have been faced with a member of your family or a friend who has unexpectedly shown an extreme form of this emotion. Mark on the mixing desk how comfortable you felt dealing with this. If you can't remember exactly, make an educated guess.

Professional Lens

Now imagine you are in a work setting. During a seemingly normal interaction that you wouldn't expect to prompt an emotional reaction, a service user suddenly displays an extreme emotion. Mark how comfortable you feel you would be in dealing with this. Think about why this would be the case.

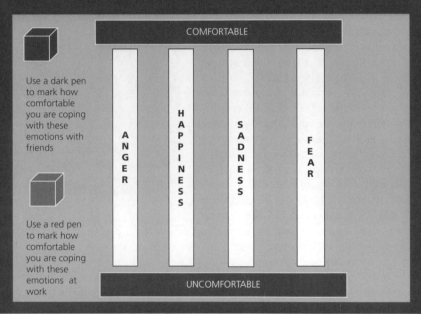

Box 5.4: Degree of comfort with emotional expression in different cultural settings

PROXEMICS (DISTANCE)

Hall was amongst the first people to recognise that space speaks to us, and that what it has to say is determined by our cultural experiences (Hall, 1966; Hall, 1959). Figure 5.2 illustrates Hall's model of distances that are frequently used within communication texts (for example Devito, 1997), and Table 5.2 identifies the characteristics of each. To accommodate the different cultural norms of this readership, a mix of imperial and metric is used!

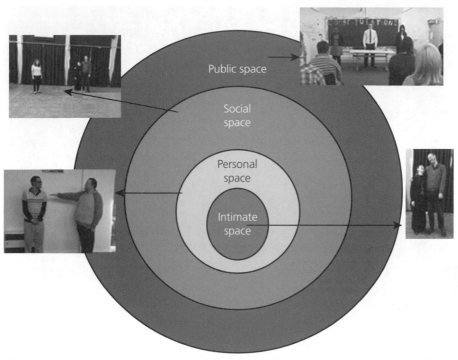

Figure 5.2: Distances and their impact upon communication (after Hall, 1966; 1959)

Table 5.2: Description of Hall's distances

Type of Distance	Close phase characteristics	Farthest phase characteristics
Public Distance (12–25 ft or more)	12 ft 3.6 m is far enough to move away in time if feeling threatened.	25 ft 7.6 m is the furthest distance from which we can effectively communicate with individuals. It is the type of distance that is granted to important public figures when at events (e.g. typical distance between audience and podium).
Social Distance (4–12 ft)	4 ft 1.2 m is the distance at which we feel most comfortable interacting with strangers at social events.	12 ft 7.6 m is the type of distance that would be maintained in the office of an important person when they interact with clients.

(Continued)

Type of Distance	Close phase characteristics	Farthest phase characteristics
Personal Distance (18 inches to 4 ft)	18 inches At 0.5 m we can reach out and touch the other person by extending an arm. We can see small details on their faces, such as lines and wrinkles. You will generally only let people you are comfortable with into this space.	4 ft At 1.2 m people can only touch if both extend their arms. This therefore determines the limit at which one person can have physical control over another. You may feel more comfortable at this distance if you have to interact but don't know the person particularly well.
Intimate Distance	6 inches 30 cm At this distance you can smell the other person, feel the heat of their body, and hear the quietest whisper. It is generally reserved for people with whom we are intimate, or for specialist sports (such as judo or wrestling).	18 inches 0.5 m This distance is uncomfortable for many people unless they are very close to the communication partner. Even if people are in a close relationship, this may feel too close in public settings.

In reality, the types of distances with which we are comfortable are determined by the cultures in which we operate, and this can create all kinds of difficulty when people from different cultures meet. For example, Hall (1959) describes a scene at a party in which someone from a Latin culture and an American culture interact. The person from the Latin culture prefers a closer social distance to the American. Every time they try to close the gap between them to accommodate this, the American backs away to recreate the distance they are comfortable with. This keeps on occurring until eventually they have crossed the room, with neither individual conscious of what is happening. However, at some level the Latin communicator may feel that the American is unfriendly, whilst the American feels the Latin communicator is overly familiar. Each judges the other in a negative light without being conscious as to why they feel that way. Communicate2U created a video to illustrate this in action and the details as to how to find it are in Box 5.6. As we have noted many times, culture is a tricky thing, and aspects of distance can be particularly hidden from us, partly because we think we know what is 'the norm'. In some cultures, being close enough to smell the other person's breath is an important part of the communication exchange, whilst in many Western cultures it would be considered impolite to, first, be that close, and second, have breath that smells (Jandt, 2007; Neuliep, 2009). Use the exercise in Box 5.5 to start to become aware of your own personal comfort zones.

Cultural norms that relate to distance do not only occur at the level of nation or ethnic origin. They are also influenced by factors such as the age of the communicators, the sex, the geographical density of the population (if there is limited living space, people get used to being closer) and the norms of the setting in which the interaction occurs (Neuliep, 2009). It is this latter factor that we will now consider in the context of health and social care interactions.

Space Invaders – Close Encounters of the Intercultural Kind

Meetings between health and social care staff and service users may be characterised by routine invasions of personal space that can make either party uncomfortable. Staff may invade service user space, and service users may invade staff space. We'll start by considering staff invasions.

Healthcare settings often involve a change in the cultural norms that we expect to occur in other aspects of our lives. For example, physical

What are your personal comfort zones?

Start to become aware of how wide your own personal boundaries are in different cultural settings. Do not use a tape measure!

Family Lens

At home having a close emotional chat with a family member or partner who needs support.

Social Group Lens

With a group of friends in a public space. Does everyone in the group maintain the same distance? What happens if you move closer to someone to chat than you normally would?

? How do you feel?

? How do they react?

Box 5.5: Personal comfort zones under the cultural lens

examinations require the staff member to come into the space that is normally reserved for those we know intimately. The member of staff is familiar with the procedure and routine, they control the situation and they get used to being close enough to touch. For the person on the receiving end of the examination, however, this can feel very threatening and intrusive. Research into the ways in which both staff and service users view gynaecological examinations has identified a range of strategies that people use to cope with actions that would normally be considered to be a gross overstepping of social rules around touch by a stranger. Staff may use set scripts that they use to depersonalise the examination and to prepare the service user for a very personal invasion of space. For example, they will explain the procedure to place the interaction within a medical context, and provide a sheet to maintain a semblance of privacy. Service users often also have coping mechanisms that allow them to view the encounter as a very specific and legitimate exception to the social norms that govern the use of personal space (Christine Edwards, 1998; Galasiński et al., 2007). Some invasions of personal space are less extreme than a gynaecological

National/Ethnic Lens

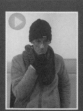

Watch the video created by Communicate2U that shows people from different national backgrounds interacting. See what happens when each tries to create a personal space that is in line with their national norm.

Social Cultural Lens

Imagine you are on your own walking along a road after a party and it is getting dark. You hear footsteps and you realise that someone is coming up behind you and getting closer and closer. You speed up – they do too. Despite there being room to avoid you, they keep on approaching – they are so close that you can hear them breathing and feel their body right next to yours ... they reach out and touch you ...

? How would you feel?

? How would you react?

? How would you then react when they handed you the keys that you had dropped? They've lost their voice and couldn't call out to you ...

Organisational Lens

Think of settings in which you as a professional may work.

? Which professions routinely invade personal space as a cultural norm?

? Are there any routines that people adopt to help make service users comfortable with this?

? Can you think of any ways in which you could reduce the risk of service users feeling and reacting as you did in the above scene?

Box 5.6: Space under the cultural lens

examination, but far more common. For example, assistance with personal care in health or care settings often involves the member of staff not only getting close to the service user, but also expecting them to be unclothed. This situation is usually only reserved for very intimate relationships. For service users who cannot understand why these norms are being challenged there is no set script that they can revert to and it can be a very frightening experience indeed. For the staff member it may be a quick routine support session, for the service user, it could be a traumatic experience akin to an assault.

Invasions of personal space have been identified as triggers for service users to exhibit behaviours that staff perceive as challenging (Ragneskog *et al.*, 1998). When people are stressed, they may require up to four times the personal space that was outlined in the diagram above (McCloskey, 2004). All of us prefer more space if we feel threatened as this gives time and space to protect ourselves. It is easy to forget that communicatively vulnerable people often feel scared in health and social care settings as they can't understand what is going on around them. Therefore, they are routinely likely to need more space to feel safe. If staff interactions are driven by the need to complete a procedural outcome and inadequate consideration is given to managing the communication elements associated with the interaction, then vulnerable services users may well react adversely. If staff realise that the zone in which service users feel safe may be as far as 25 feet, and start to use non-verbal strategies to indicate that they are non-threatening from this distance, they may find that the risk of precipitating an incident is reduced. Have a go at the exercise in Box 5.6; think about the settings in which you as a professional may work, and how routine invasions of space may be managed. Use the information on non-verbal behaviour within this chapter to help you.

It is not only service users who may experience discomfort at the invasion of personal space in the work setting. Staff too may experience this as they meet people from a range of different cultural backgrounds who habitually prefer a different personal space than is the Western norm. It may occur with people from different national or ethnic backgrounds, or with service users who may be vulnerable in communication exchanges. Service users may have conditions in which it is not uncommon for personal space boundaries to be set at distances which conflict with the national norm – for example, learning disability or autistic spectrum disorder (Eigsti *et al.*, 2011), schizophrenia (Park *et al.*, 2009) or dementia (McCloskey, 2004; Moyle *et al.*, 2008). They may come too close and invade staff space, or stand at a distance which may unconsciously make staff move closer, which creates a threat to which the service user reacts. Either distance conflicts with staff cultural norms and creates a feeling of discomfort. Misinterpreting non-verbal behaviour as hostile and stereotyping the other as being the person who is at fault is characteristic of intercultural conflict (Barna, 1997). Recognising that the other person may have a different set of rules that govern their use of personal space, and that we are feeling uncomfortable because it conflicts with our own (usually hidden) cultural rules is an important first step in making the encounter more comfortable. The exercises in this section have been designed to help you start to develop this awareness and will hopefully make it easier to also develop an intercultural perspective of the skills that we will focus on in the following section: movements and gesture (kinesics).

MOVEMENT AND GESTURE (KINESICS)

Take a look at the two pictures below and decide which person you would feel more comfortable communicating with:

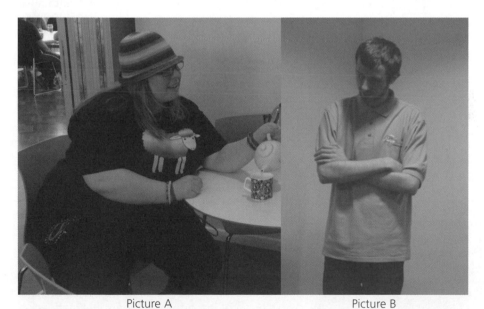

Picture A   Picture B

Figure 5.3: Open and closed body language

You are probably familiar with the concept that open body language, characterised by head up, arms relaxed and uncrossed (picture A) facilitates communication whilst closed body language (picture B) closes it down. However, you may not fully realise the degree to which this dominates communication with people who do not have easy access to words. For some service users, the words that are used to accompany body language comes across as meaningless noise; they are focusing not on *what* you say, but *how* you say it (Cascella, 2005; Kacperek, 1997; Stephenson *et al.*, 2005). The words convey the facts, but the body movements communicate our thoughts and feelings. Health and social care training often includes consideration as to how to manage body language in specific circumstances (such as giving bad news) (Silverman *et al.*, 1998; Volker *et al.*, 2004) but in fact our bodies are sending messages about our emotional state to service users and carers every time that we meet them. The degree to which we are conscious of this and control the movement of our bodies varies according to the type of movement concerned (Devito, 1997). In the sections below we will consider different types of movements in the context of different cultures.

EMBLEMS

Emblems are movements that can be directly translated into words (Devito, 1997). At some level we know and understand that these gestures are symbolic. The movements are generally learned in the same way that we learn a language – through informal learning (Hall, 1959), and they therefore have a strong cultural component (Neuliep, 2009). Some examples of emblems are shown in Table 5.3.

As culture is generally hidden from us, it can be a shock to learn that some of these seemingly innocent gestures are actually considered very insulting in other parts of the world. (We will leave it up to you to explore the many meanings associated with them – thank you Internet search engines!) Cultural use of emblems also occurs in social groups and families. Have a go at the exercise in Box 5.7 to develop your awareness of emblems in these cultures.

Within health and social care settings, specific cultural groups may develop specialised use of emblems. Staff may know what particular gestures represent and this knowledge may be hidden from service users who are unfamiliar with the setting. However, service users and carers may also have knowledge of important emblems that staff lack.

Some service users such as those with hearing impairment or learning disability may make use of language systems that are primarily based on gesture (for example sign language or Makaton). In such cases, the service user, family or carer will

---

Emblems

Social Lens

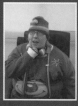

Have a look at a sports match on TV and note how many emblems you can spot being used by players and spectators during the game.

Family Lens

Amy and Janet had a friend Emily who tended to over indulge, then complain that she didn't understand why she was putting weight on. One day, whilst she was making this comment she left the room and Amy puffed out her cheeks to indicate 'not the same old story!' Janet interpreted this as 'she's really fat!' and when they realised their mistakes, both fell about laughing. From then on, puffing out the cheeks was always their private gesture to indicate that they were talking about Emily.

Do you have any emblems that are specific to your family or friends?

Box 5.7: Emblems under the cultural lens

Table 5.3: Common emblems and their meanings

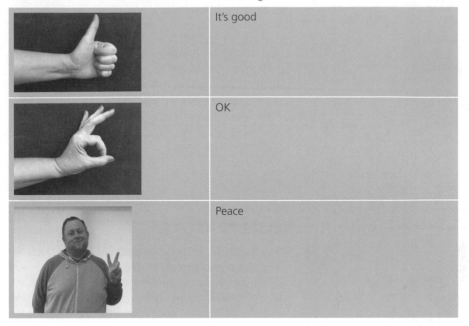	It's good
	OK
	Peace

be the cultural experts, and the staff member is the less competent communicator. What may appear to be a casual, unimportant movement may actually be a very specific request. For example, a person with a learning disability who is flicking their hand across their shoulder is asking for the toilet, and may become very distressed if they are not shown where it is very quickly. It would be unrealistic to expect all health and social care staff to learn all the potential languages that they are likely to encounter. However, we argue here that just as it is polite to learn a few basic words in a foreign country in which you are holidaying, it is vital to learn a few basic phrases that belong to the most vulnerable communicators in health and social care settings. Communicate2U developed a song to help you to learn some of the basics. Look at the information in Box 5.8 and learn from the cultural experts.

Communication passports and toolkits can act as dictionaries to help bridge the communication gap, but they are only going to be used if staff recognise that gestures such as those shown above are forms of symbolic communication that they need to learn. Failing to recognise these

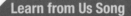
Learn from Us Song

Communicate2U have written a song to help you learn some basic Makaton and to remember simple rules for communicating with vulnerable people.

Feedback from students and staff indicates that this has been a highly effective method of learning and retaining the information.

Please take the time to look at the online video and join in trying out the Makaton symbols. The last chorus is repeated to help reinforce your learning.

Box 5.8: Learn from us – Communicate2U teach basic communication skills and Makaton in a song

Illustrators

Have a go at performing the following interactions by using body movements (either in pairs, or by imagining that you are with another person).

Verbal message	Body Movement
Please sit down	Points to chair
Go straight along this corridor	Point down the corridor
Do you want a drink?	Mime a cup at the lips
The dog was huge!	Use hands to illustrate the height, length and width of the animal

How often do you tend to use these types of gestures when speaking?

? **The next time that you're at a social gathering, look around and start to notice how much other people use their bodies to support the verbal message. Do some people use more movements than others?**

Now consider your work role and the types of messages you frequently need to convey. Are there some gestures that could be used to illustrate these messages to make them more accessible to people who find words and concepts hard to understand? An example has been given to start you off.

Verbal Message	Body Movement
Let's get dressed	Points to clothes on the chair
	Holds first item up
	Mimes putting on a garment
	Hands garment to person

Box 5.9: Use of illustrators in different cultural groups

types of gestures as language can lead to communicatively vulnerable service users becoming malnourished (Iacono *et al.*, 2003), dehydrated (Cumella *et al.*, 2004), suffering unnecessary pain (Michael *et al.*, 2008) or social isolation (Finlay *et al.*, 2007). Increasing your awareness of how you use emblems across all of your cultural settings, and recognising that these may be a primary form of communication for people who have an awareness of symbolism (but difficulties using words) should help to reduce the risk of this form of communication being overlooked in health and care settings.

ILLUSTRATORS

Illustrators are the natural movements that accompany our communication (Devito, 1997). They are not as symbolic as emblems (although they are still somewhat removed from the actual object or concept itself), and therefore have less of a cultural component. However, there may still be some cultural variation (Ekman, 1976). For example, if someone is describing a tall person, they may raise their hand to the approximate height to help illustrate the verbal message. This is likely to be understood across cultures; if you are asked by a foreigner to give directions, you are very likely to use a lot of pointing in different directions to accompany your description. There may be some innate component to basic illustrators (Argyle, 2013; Bull, 1983), and so this may help to make it easier for people who find words hard to understand the verbal message. Although there is less of a cultural component to decoding this type of message, the degree to which different cultures use illustrators may vary. People from Latin cultures, for example, tend to use a greater number of gestures to accompany speech than those from Western cultures (Jandt, 2007). People who find words or symbolic use of emblems difficult may still benefit from the clues that more natural illustrators give them. However, if you don't naturally use this form of communication in your home or social cultural groups, you may not naturally use them in the work setting unless you start to become consciously aware of this as a communication skill. Have a go at the exercise in Box 5.9 to explore how comfortable you are with using illustrators in your different cultural groups, and how you could use these types of gestures to illustrate the messages that you often try to convey in your professional role.

AFFECT DISPLAYS AND EYE CONTACT

Affect displays are those body movements that directly convey the emotional message. They therefore are non-symbolic and are produced by everyone (Devito, 1997). This concept has already been discussed in the section on facial expression, and you will therefore be familiar with the idea that basic emotions are recognised across cultures. Here we will explore how the rest of the body sends out this type of emotional message.

We are often quite conscious of the message that our face needs to send within a given cultural setting and we attend to our facial expression when we consciously want to create an impression. However, unless the whole body is giving the same message then we may give away our true feelings. For example, when going for a job interview, we know that we need to smile when we greet the interviewer to appear confident and pleasant, but if the rest of our body language is shouting that we are very nervous, then this is the message that is likely to be listened to. Figure 5.4 illustrates this point.

The tension within our muscles, the degree to which our body is orientated towards the communication partner and the angle at which our head is held (to give but a few examples) all serve to show our degree of interest in the communication partner, and how comfortable we are at communicating with them. If the focus is on the verbal message, then this type of communication can be overlooked. We only see what we are culturally conditioned to see, and this point leads us to the importance of eye contact and gaze within communication exchanges.

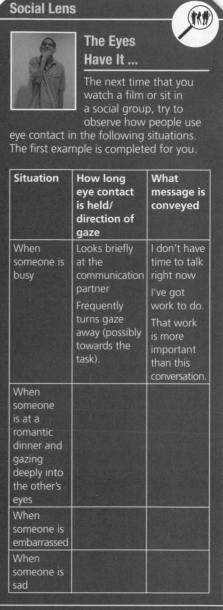

Social Lens

The Eyes Have It ...

The next time that you watch a film or sit in a social group, try to observe how people use eye contact in the following situations. The first example is completed for you.

Situation	How long eye contact is held/ direction of gaze	What message is conveyed
When someone is busy	Looks briefly at the communication partner. Frequently turns gaze away (possibly towards the task).	I don't have time to talk right now. I've got work to do. That work is more important than this conversation.
When someone is at a romantic dinner and gazing deeply into the other's eyes		
When someone is embarrassed		
When someone is sad		

Box 5.10: Eye contact in different settings

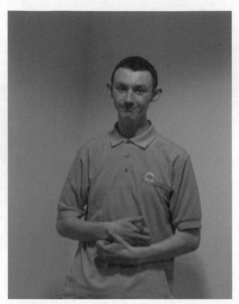

Figure 5.4: Picture illustrating a nervous smile

Eye contact is regarded by some researchers as the most important of all message systems, without which people do not feel that they are fully communicating (Argyle *et al.*, 1965; Hargie *et al.*, 1997). It has a number of functions including:

- Seeking feedback from others
- Regulating the conversation (helping to indicate whose turn it is to communicate)
- Signalling the relationship between the communicators (the longing look, or the disdainful glance)
- Bringing communicators closer together even though the physical distance may be large (think of catching someone's eye across a crowded room) (Knapp *et al.*, 2013)

Eye contact is an innate form of communication amongst all people who have vision. Some of the earliest forms of communication that most humans experience come in the form of eye contact between infant and caregiver. This process forms the basis of the communicative bond that later evolves into more sophisticated forms of communication (Trevarthen, 1979). The rules that then develop around the use of eye contact are influenced by culture, and therefore it has been said that mother culture develops before mother-tongue (Bullowa, 1979). Since the rules are cultural in nature, they are generally hidden from those people that use them (Hall, 1959), but the message conveyed by the duration, direction and quality of eye movement is very powerful. For example, in the UK and USA, the average length of gaze before someone looks away from another person is 2.95 seconds, and if both happen to look at each other at the same time, this drops to around 1.18 seconds. Looking at someone for less time is interpreted to mean disinterest or shyness, whilst a longer gaze is perceived as unusually high interest (Devito, 1997). Direct eye contact is considered a sign of honesty, and people who avoid this are generally considered to be devious (Beebe, 1974). People who are adept at managing their image (such as politicians or business people) may therefore consciously attempt to hold another's gaze whilst lying (Burns *et al.*, 1976). However, in many cultures, direct eye contact is considered disrespectful, or an indication that the communication partner is of the same status (Jandt, 2007). Failing to recognise cultural differences in the cultural rules that govern eye contact can therefore lead to some serious misunderstandings; an English business partner may judge a Japanese customer who looks away to be untrustworthy, whilst the Japanese business partner feels they are showing respect. As in previous sections, the key to avoiding these types of misunderstandings is acknowledging that miscommunication may be cultural in nature, and trying to avoid a stance of cultural superiority (Barna, 1997).

Service users in health and social care settings may have different cultural norms that govern their use of eye contact. People on the autistic spectrum (Farroni *et al.*, 2002; Senju *et al.*, 2009), people with a learning disability (Bradley *et al.*, 2005; Eigsti *et al.*, 2011), dementia (Feil, 2014) or schizophrenia (Kington *et al.*, 2000), to name just a few examples, often have an average length of gaze that is different to the cultural norm. Staff may therefore feel very uncomfortable and threatened because they interpret a prolonged gaze as hostile or overly familiar, or a shorter gaze as disinterested. Service users and families too experience discomfort when staff violate their cultural norms. In families with good communication there is an expectation that staff should speak to and look at the service user who is the subject of an intervention or discussion. However, health and social care staff often do not look at service users who have limited or absent verbal communication (McConkey *et al.*, 1999), and they frequently direct their communication straight to the carer (Finlay *et al.*, 2007; Iacono *et al.*, 2003). This violates a very profound cultural norm. In Western cultures, looking at an individual gives them status as a communication partner (Mehrabian, 1969; Mehrabian, 1971). Overlooking communicatively vulnerable people therefore denies them access to status as a communicating human being. Small wonder that service users and family members or carers find this so distressing, as Sadie illustrated in her quotation (Communicate2U Quote 3.1) in Chapter 3. Increasing cultural sensitivity to the importance of eye contact can help to improve interactions between people from different cultural backgrounds.

A person on the autistic spectrum who looks away whilst thinking (Senju *et al.*, 2009) is exhibiting the same type of cultural eye contact strategies as someone from Japan. All of us will have had times in our lives outside of work when we have chosen to look away from a communication partner. Eye avoidance is a strategy that those in Western cultures routinely use to show that we are respecting privacy, or to shut out distractions so we can concentrate better (Devito, 1997; Goffman, 1967). We may shut our eyes to concentrate on a piece of music. Many people close their eyes whilst kissing a lover. We would not automatically assume that the Japanese person or the lover should be excluded from a communication exchange, and we would not consider ourselves to be incompetent communicators because we avoid gaze when listening to music at a concert or kissing. However, there may be a tendency to make these types of assumptions within health and social care settings when we meet people who use gaze differently. Use the exercises in Box 5.10 to explore your own cultural norms that relate to eye contact and gaze and to become more aware of the ways in which others do the same. If you are prepared for the discomfort that different use of eye contact may cause you, but are capable of seeing this as a cultural difference to which you need to adapt, you are more likely to make use of this vital component of body movement. This can help you to become a more effective health or social care professional (Mast, 2007).

REGULATORS

Regulators are the movements (and sounds) that we use to try to control the person who is interacting with us (Devito, 1997). For example, if we wish some-one to continue talking, we may nod and smile to encourage them. If we want them to let us have a turn, we may raise our eyes and open our mouths as if ready to speak to give them a sign that they should yield he conversation to us. All of these cues are culture specific, none of them are written down as specific rules, and therefore they can be misinterpreted by people who have different cultural backgrounds. If someone ignores our cues the usual response is to assume that they are rude (Barna, 1997), whereas they may just be following their own cultural norms. Staff in health and social care settings often have spe-cific outcomes that they want to achieve within a short space of time, and may use regulators to try to control the interaction to fit. People who are vulnerable communicators may need to have the boundaries for the interaction clearly laid out as they may not pick up on regulators that would normally support turn tak-ing. Setting out what will happen during the interaction (preferably including a visual prompt for each stage of the encounter) and using statements such as 'it's your turn', 'it's my turn', or 'we're going to finish now' may make it much easier for each party to understand the hidden cultural rules that you wish someone to follow.

ADAPTORS

Adaptors are movements that we engage in when we respond to an inner drive (Devito, 1997). For example, we feel an itch and respond to it by scratching ourselves, or we wriggle because we are becoming uncomfortable. The move-ments therefore convey a message about our needs. We will all perform some of these movements unconsciously (for example when we move during our sleep), but may be aware of cultural norms that prevent us from performing the movements in public (for example, scratching one's bottom in front of others). The type of information that is included on communication passports or the Disability Distress Assessment Tool (DisDAT) (Regnard et al., 2007) could be considered as the means by which the families and carers of people with high communication needs translate their knowledge of adaptor movements into a word-based format that is accessible to health and social care staff. Passports in paper (Thurman et al., 2005) or electronic formats (Bradshaw, 2013) are therefore actually the distilled knowledge of many months or years of cultural experience. Those health and social care staff who view this knowledge with cultural respect have access to the key to decode information about the needs of the most vulnerable people with whom they work.

TOUCH (HAPTICS)

Touch is one of the most primitive and powerful ways in which meaning can be communicated. Stimulation from touch starts in the womb, and the degree and type of handling that an infant receives can have a lasting impact upon emotional, intellectual and physiological development (Andersen et al., 1978; Fisher et al., 1976). Touch can communicate basic emotional messages, but, possibly because it is so powerful, the cultural rules that govern its use can differ widely. Devito (1997) identifies five major meanings that are communicated by touch:

1. **Positive emotions:** affection, support and trust can be communicated by actions such as a hug or a touch on the shoulder or the hand. In health and social care settings, positive touch has been shown to facilitate self-disclosure (Pattison, 1973) and verbalisation (Willis Jr et al., 1980).
2. **Playfulness:** we may communicate an intention to play, or to say something in a playful mood through our use of touch. For example, a jokey statement may be accompanied by a light tap that tells the other person that you are not serious.
3. **Control:** touch can be used to move another person, to gain their attention, or to dominate them.
4. **Ritual:** many greetings are accompanied by some degree of touch – for example, a handshake or kiss on the cheek at the start of an interaction (depending on culture). The example of an examination used earlier in this chapter could also be considered as a highly specialised ritual form of touch that occurs within a culture. It is ritualised in that it is performed in the same way each time. However, it could also be considered to be part of the next category:
5. **Task Related:** Some tasks such as helping someone out of a chair naturally have an element of touch if they are to be completed.

Categorising touch in this way actually hides much of the complexity that governs its use. For each of these categories, the degree to which each person

Touch under the cultural lens

How comfortable are you with touch?

Have a look at the following cultural settings and decide how comfortable you are with touching/being touched in each of them.

Social Group Cultural Lens You are introduced to someone for the first time in a social situation (such as a party)	Do you use touch to initiate the greeting (e.g. a handshake or kiss on the cheek)? Do you prefer to only use words? If someone goes to greet you with a kiss on the cheek, how do you feel?
Family Cultural Lens Somebody is upset in your family and needs comfort	Would you use touch to comfort them? How and where would you touch them? What factors may influence your decision?
Professional Lens A service user is with you and starts to cry	Would you use touch to comfort them? How and where would you touch them? What factors may influence your decision? Are there any guidelines on the therapeutic use of touch in your profession?

Box 5.11: Use of touch in different cultural settings

within the interaction feels the touch is acceptable will vary upon a wide number of additional factors such as:

● The gender of the people interacting (same sex or opposite sex)
● The age of the people concerned
● How well the people know each other
● The roles that each person occupies
● The setting in which the touch occurs
● What part of the body is touched and for how long
● Explicit cultural rules about touch
● Personal views about touch

In many cultures there are cultural taboos against a stranger touching an individual, and a violation of these norms can be extremely distressing. For example, people from Japan are likely to find touch from a stranger much more intrusive that people from Latin America. Alongside the cultural rules governing touch there is also a strong personal component to the degree to which we are comfortable with touching others and being touched ourselves. Have a go at the exercise in Box 5.11 to explore how comfortable you are with touch in different cultural settings.

In health and social care settings touch could be considered as occurring for two main reasons: **instrumental touch** to carry out a procedure, and **emotional touch** (McCann et al., 1993). The types of touch used by staff will vary depending on the needs of the service user and setting. It may include the need to carry out necessary procedures that are painful, or in the case of behaviours that are perceived to be challenging, may also include the use of restraint. Although the intent of the touch is instrumental, there may well be an emotional impact on the person who is at the receiving end. For example, people with a learning disability (Dobson et al., 2002) and the elderly (McCann et al., 1993) may have had negative experiences of touch in the past and be fearful when going into situations which seem similar. Staff too may be fearful of touching as the ethical considerations are numerous and complex including as they do the potential for touch to be considered as sexual in nature (Aquino *et al.*, 2000) or an abuse of power. Whilst there may be professional guidelines that define what types of touch should be used and in what circumstances, in practice the ways in which these are implemented may vary from setting to setting and person to person, even in the same locality (Susan *et al.*, 2004). However, given that touch is a powerful communication tool, it may be an important means of communicating at an emotional level with people who find other forms of communication inaccessible. To deny this form of communication may exclude some of the most vulnerable communicators from the support that they require. The balance between protecting vulnerable service users and facilitating appropriate communication is a delicate and complex issue. The examples in Box 5.12 are drawn from the experiences of Communicate2U and reflect the difficulties that both staff and service users face in trying to negotiate the norms of touch in different settings. From an intercultural perspective, it is important to recognise that there may be an imbalance between the amount of written material on the use of touch that is produced by professionals and the amount that is produced by communicatively vulnerable individuals. Organisations and professional cultures are likely to have a range of policies, procedures and research that guide the use of touch. These will usually have been written to protect both service users and staff members, but they will have been written by members of a word-dominated culture. Service users who are communicatively vulnerable may have different expectations about the use of touch. This may be available in written format for staff to access. Communication passports, for example, may give staff clues as to what touch is acceptable and welcomed, and what kind of touch may be particularly challenging. Other service users may not have formal written documents to support them in communicating how they generally use and experience touch. Asking the service user or family about their wishes regarding touch may help to ensure that the communicative needs of vulnerable people are weighed against the needs of the organisation.

Scene 1

 An elderly man with dementia is living in a care home. He has very limited verbal understanding and becomes very distressed and tearful. A new member of staff wishes to comfort him and puts her arm around him. A more established member of staff notices this and intervenes, stating that this level of contact is against the policy of the care home. The man is led to the privacy of his bedroom to calm down privately.

Scene 2

A young man with a learning disability is waiting in an accident and emergency unit for treatment. He is becoming distressed and wants to talk to someone. He sees a person in a uniform hurrying past and grasps their arm to stop them so that he can ask a question. The staff member calls security to assist with an assault.

Looking at both scenes, consider the following points:

? **What cultural norms of touch were being challenged?**

? **Why do you think that staff responded in the way described?**

? **Do you think that the staff concerned may have responded differently had the touch occurred in their family setting?**

? **How else could they have reacted?**

Box 5.12: Implications of touch and clashing cultural norms

CHAPTER SUMMARY

That body language is powerful and important should be no surprise to prac-titioners in health and social care. Many of the components – touch, distance, facial expression and use of gesture, for example – are likely to have been a part of professional training. They are things that we consciously attend to when things are important to us: at interviews, during dates or when preparing peo-ple for bad news. However, within this chapter we have identified that many health and social care staff often feel ill-equipped to communicate with people for whom body language is a primary means of interacting with others. They think that communication with people with additional needs is difficult and they are often afraid to try. However, you have the necessary skills to see and respond to emotional communication in other cultural settings in which you interact – in your families and your social groups. You can use these same skills at work to see the emotional message that service users are communicating through their body language. You can use gesture and facial expressions to reinforce verbal mes-sages, and can consciously attend to the emotional message that your body is sending during interactions. This will increase the chances of you interacting in a meaningful and reciprocal way with people who are otherwise communicatively vulnerable.

EASY READ CHAPTER SUMMARY

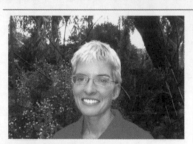

Happy

Our faces and bodies can tell other people how we are feeling

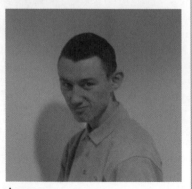

Angry

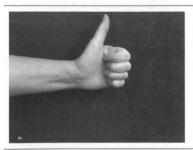

We can use our bodies to give people other messages too – like 'it's good!'

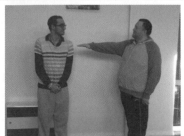

We all like to keep some space for ourselves

We can feel uncomfortable if others come too close

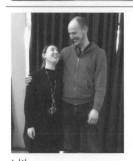

I like you

Sometimes we use touch to tell people things

When we use our bodies to say things it is called **body language**

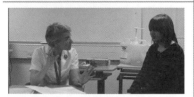

Staff who work in hospitals or homes need to be good at body language

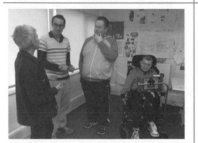

If they aren't, they may not be good at working with people who find words hard

People who find words hard may get left out and be sad, hungry or thirsty

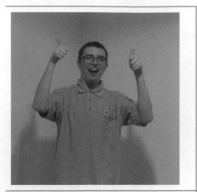

We all use body language to communicate – so it's easy!

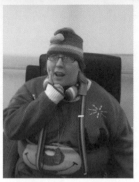

But staff need to remember to do it

ENVIRONMENTAL ASPECTS OF COMMUNICATION

By the end of this chapter you will be able to:

➡ Explain how environments affect our communication and communicate with us

➡ Analyse the concept of territoriality and apply it to cultures within which you communicate

➡ Identify the role that objects have in communicating values and messages

➡ Examine how sensory input is an intrinsic aspect of communication

➡ Identify how you can alter your work environment to improve communication with vulnerable people

INTRODUCTION

This is the final chapter in the trilogy that has focused upon non-verbal aspects of communication and it will focus upon how the environment sends messages for us to interpret and react to. The term 'environment' can be defined in a multitude of different ways, but for the purposes of this chapter we will be focusing upon the physical environment – manmade or natural objects and features that can be touched and seen. Other environmental components such as the cultural or social environment (Kielhofner, 2008) are an intrinsic part of all of the chapters in this book and will not be considered separately. The virtual environment is becoming an increasingly important component of modern day life with its own evolving communication culture and style (Biocca et al., 2013), but encounters within this realm are outside the scope of this book.

Our physical environments are the backdrop against which all of our interactions occur. This chapter will argue that all aspects of it are culturally determined and therefore many issues related to communication will be hidden from those who are members of the culture. These hidden features, however, play a very important role in communication. We take for granted that our buildings will have a certain style or shape, that objects that perform a function will have a particular look, and we learn to filter out familiar smells and sounds so that they become unimportant features that we barely notice any more. However, these seemingly boring features tell us about the values of the people who have structured the environment, and they cue us in to culturally determined patterns of behaving and communicating. For example, a library that is filled with shelves containing books and small spaces with tables and chairs gives those who are familiar with this environment an instruction: 'This is a place for reading or study. Speak quietly and don't disturb others around you.' Someone who enters the library and who does not follow these (often hidden) rules soon finds that they are considered rude and are shushed or given harsh looks. This chapter will look at how environments trigger communicative behaviour within a cultural context. By understanding the power of the environment in a range of cultures within which you operate you will be able to apply this knowledge to your workplace and adapt the environment to better meet the needs of people who are communicatively vulnerable. The elements that will be examined are shown in the table below, and as with previous chapters you are reminded that whilst we consider these separately, they are linked to all other aspects of communication.

Table 6.1: How chapters link within this book: Chapter 6

Chapter 3: Word-Based Interpersonal Communication	Chapter 4: Musical Aspects of Communication	Chapter 5: Body Language	Chapter 6: Environmental Aspects of Communication	Chapter 7: Professional Scripts
• The role of words • Inclusive and exclusive communication • Scripting	• Pitch/Key • Vocal qualifiers • Volume • Pace/Rate/Timing • Silence	• Proxemics (distance) • Kinesics (movements and gesture) • Haptics (touch) • Facial expression	• **Physical environment** • **Objects** • **Territoriality** • **Sensory input as communication**	• Putting the chapters together to perform your role

TERRITORIALITY AND POWER

Like many animals, humans are territorial beings (Devito, 1997), and like many animals the size and nature of the territory that we inhabit is linked to our status (Mehrabian, 1971). However, unlike animals, whose actions are driven by biology, human territoriality can be viewed as being driven more by socially constructed rules that determine the amount and type of space that an individual or group are permitted to occupy (Sack, 1986). Those with the most power tend have the most choice as to which spaces they lay claim to. People in authority have the nicest offices or desks, and the higher up the power chain you go the more likely it is that you will be in an imposing building in the most expensive part of town. This reflects the ease with which people can access resources such as money (exclusive parts of town are limited in space and cost more), status, and control of the agenda relating to resource allocation. If you need to refresh your memory on the types of power that people have, go back to Chapter 2. Whatever position we occupy in the hierarchy, most of us will try to exert influence to have some control over the space around us. This may be a conscious or an unconscious process. In his study of institutions, Goffman (1961) observed that a more communicatively able patient in a mental institution was very effective at selecting the most comfortable chair and was able to drive off a non-verbal patient who briefly tried to lay claim to it. Although the patient was relatively disempowered in nearly every other aspect of his life, his ability to communicate with words gave him power over territory. This chapter will start by looking at how the spaces that we occupy link to communication in our different cultural settings.

TERRITORY

Territory is defined here as the spaces over which we exert control, and **territoriality** is defined as the behaviours that we engage in to defend those spaces. Territory can be categorised in different ways, and some theorists would include the space that we considered in Chapter 5 under the heading of proxemics as being body territory and a category in its own right (Lyman *et al.*, 1967). However, here we will consider territory in terms of primary, secondary and public (Altman, 1975) and relate this to some of the settings in which health and social care staff and communicatively vulnerable people interact.

Primary Territory

Primary territory is ours. It is the place that we control and that we defend if it is invaded. It is usually the place in which we feel safe, and we take the lead in interactions. We have power in this space and feel more dominant, even if a person who is usually more powerful than us enters it. It is our bedroom at home, our car or the home ground of our football team, for example. The space affects the way that we feel and the ways in which we communicate. For example, when we

Territory, Role and Power

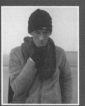

Have a look at the list of people below. What kind of room do you imagine them in when you read the word?

- Rock stars
- Politicians
- Students
- Professional health and social care staff
- People on benefits
- Children

Now think about the territories that you enter in your own life. As you look at the list of these shown below, think of the following:

? **What do these spaces mean to you?**

? **How do you feel when you are in them?**

? **How happy are you for strangers to enter them?**

? **Does your communication style vary between spaces?**

Primary Territory (Family Lens)

Bedroom at home

Secondary (Organisational Lens)

Work or study space

Public (Social Group Lens)

Your local park or shopping centre

Box 6.1: Your territory in different cultural settings

are in a primary territory, we are more likely to initiate an interaction, have an informal conversational style and dominate an interaction, regardless of who we are communicating with (Marsh, 1988). We also unconsciously or consciously set the rules for that space: we decide whether people should take their shoes off before entering our house, for example, and whether it is appropriate for them to sit on a particular chair. Have a go at the exercise in Box 6.1 to explore how you feel about your territories in different cultural settings and how you communicate in each.

As health and social care staff we meet service users in a variety of settings. Sometimes we will do home visits in which we enter someone else's primary territory. As we step over the threshold, some of our power is diminished: the service user knows the rules of the house, and we do not. If we do not adhere to the cultural expectations associated with that territory, we are likely to set the scene for difficulties within the interaction as shown in the case study example in Box 6.2. Have a go at trying to work out why Mrs Eckmann was unhappy:

Mrs Eckmann had been an inpatient in hospital for some weeks and was now ready for discharge. She needed a home visit from the occupational therapist to determine what equipment would be required. She and the therapist had developed a good rapport and both were looking forward to the visit as being the final stage of recovery. As they arrived, Mrs Eckmann slipped off her shoes and went into the house. The therapist followed and both started to go through assessments of everyday tasks. Mrs Eckmann became increasingly short tempered as the visit progressed, and whereas before she had welcomed suggestions from the therapist, was now starting to question why some of the suggested ideas were needed. The therapist recognised the change in mood and asked if anything was worrying her about her return home. She replied shortly that she was fine. The atmosphere during the visit was decidedly frosty, and both were glad when it was over.

Box 6.2: Case Scenario: Territorial issues when a therapist enters a service user's home

In the above case scenario, Mrs Eckmann had had a new carpet delivered shortly before being admitted into hospital. She was very house proud and kept an immaculate home. She expected all visitors to remove footwear to keep it that way, but felt unable to ask the therapist to do so as they had developed a relationship in which she followed the therapist's lead. She expected the therapist to see how she took her shoes off and follow her lead now that she was in her own place. The therapist had seen her do this, but her health and safety regulations for home visits required her to keep her own shoes on at all times to prevent injury. As she kept her shoes on in her own home, she did not see how important this was to Mrs Eckmann, and attributed her change in mood to nerves about the forthcoming discharge. As Mrs Eckmann was now in her own territory, she felt more confident about expressing her displeasure with disapproving body language and tone of voice, even if she did not feel confident enough to say something explicitly.

When entering someone else's home, health and social care staff need to be conscious of the fact that power dynamics will have shifted. Failing to acknowledge the shift in power towards the service user may cause interpersonal communication to be more difficult than it needs to be. It is highly unlikely that many of the rules of the territory will be made explicit to health and social care staff. They will be communicated through the environment in the form of decorations or objects (as we will explore later in this chapter). However, if staff can pick up on these cues to respect the values of the service user, then communication may be even more effective since the individual is more likely to be relaxed and able to communicate in a way that they feel comfortable with. In many cases, service users are expected to enter territories in which health and social care staff are more dominant – the territory of the work place. An office that is assigned to us on a long term basis can be considered to be a primary territory. Many people, however, have less permanent arrangements and the workspace may then fall under the heading of a secondary territory.

Secondary Territory

Secondary territories do not belong to us, but they are ones with which we feel an affinity. They often occur in places which we regularly inhabit such as a café, place of study or work place. For example, it may be a bay in a clinic or a meeting room that we use on a regular basis, or a chair in a classroom in which we habitually sit. Mrs Eckman's story in Box 6.2 illustrated how the style of communication is affected by territory. She was in control in her own home (primary territory) and therefore felt less constrained. The type of territory can also affect the form of communication used. This can be illustrated by considering our secondary territories: desks or offices. For example, the way that people communicate at work will be affected by whether their desk is one that is permanently assigned, or whether they have to go to whichever is available (a hot desk). Employees that use hot desks are more likely to use electronic means (such as email) to communicate with colleagues. Those with a fixed desk tend to talk to people more (Millward *et al.*, 2007). There are therefore some powerful and hidden cultural aspects to communication at work (pun intended!), whether the secondary territory is a desk, clinical area, or other official work space. Although there is no formal ownership of the secondary space, we feel an attachment to it and may get upset if others sit in our chair or at our desk, even if they have a right to do so (Devito, 1997).

Health and social care staff have control over their secondary territories and can determine the communication form and style that they use with service users when they interact in those spaces. When you are in your usual place of work you are more relaxed than service users and will be more dominant. Service users may react to this dominance in a range of ways, but for this section we will confine the discussion to those that conform to the expectations that you hold for the territory, and those who don't. Service users who conform to your expectations will generally be those who understand the hidden rules that such spaces carry with them: the ones who believe that you are a professional, that you are there to support them and that what you say or do is in their best interests. They may find it difficult to express their real feelings and thoughts in case

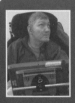

How do you expect service users to behave in your work space?

? Who decides where they should sit?

? Who starts the discussion or interaction?

? Is the communication style formal or informal?

? Who decides what form of communication takes place? E.g. Spoken word, written communication, pictures or Makaton?

? Who decides the content of the discussion – you or the service user?

How do you feel when service users don't behave in the way that you expect? Have a look at the points below and answer honestly.

A service user who you have never met before comes and sits in your spot without you asking them to.

? What may be the first thing that goes through your mind?

? How could you react?

Box 6.3: Territory, feelings and communicating with service users

they overstep some hidden boundary. Those who don't conform to these expectations are breaking some of the territorial rules that you will have consciously or unconsciously set and you may feel uncomfortable. Have a go at the exercise in Box 6.3 to explore what your expectations in this territory are.

Public Territory

Public territories are spaces that everyone can access (Altman, 1975; Devito, 1997). They may be parks, libraries, concert halls or shopping centres. Each can be considered as a cultural environment in their own right that has its own set of rules of behaviour and expectations regarding how people communicate. Some of the rules may be written down (for example, don't step on the grass), and some may be assumed but never written (for example, don't bring your washing to dry in the public park). As public spaces do not imply a difference in power relations between people who informally occupy them, they may be useful spaces for some interactions between health and social care staff and service users. For example, people who feel disempowered may be overawed by the formality of a work space, but may feel more able to relax and discuss important issues with health or social care staff in a garden or café area.

TERRITORIALITY

Territories are important. They are not neutral spaces, but are areas in which we express our personalities and values. They carry a personal meaning and it is therefore not surprising that we can get upset if others enter those spaces and do not respect the things that we feel are important. Lyman and Scott (1967) identified three key ways in which others can encroach upon our territory:

1. Violation
2. Invasion
3. Contamination

Violation occurs when another individual or group enters a territory and uses it in such a way as to alter the meaning of that territory for the person who normally occupies that space. The therapist in Box 6.2 did that when she rendered the pristine home environment dirty in the eyes of the home owner.

Invasion occurs when another enters the territory and lays claim to the space. Examples of invasion can be seen on public beaches where holiday makers have attempted to make an area of sand their own (perhaps by using towels), and others come and move the towels to make space for their deck chairs. People from different national cultures have different norms about what is acceptable in such situations, which can lead to some quite heated exchanges as neither party recognises that different cultural values are in play and assumes that the other is aggressively invading their space (Smith, 1981).

Contamination occurs when a territory is rendered impure (Devito, 1997). For example, someone with an intense dislike of dirt has a visitor who sits on their chair with mud splattered jeans. The chair cannot be used again until it has been purified by washing with disinfectant (or in extreme cases it may be replaced). Contamination requires an act of purification before the territory can feel the same again.

When we feel that our territory has been threatened in the ways that are described above, we naturally want to react to minimise the threat to our space and the values that are associated with it. One of the ways that we do this is to erect barriers to show others what our space is – a process known as **insulation** (Devito, 1997). These may be physical barriers such as fences; objects that limit communication (such as an actor wearing sunglasses in public); and communicative barriers. **Linguistic collusion** – using professional jargon that others cannot understand – can help us to erect barriers between ourselves and those who are not part of the profession (Devito, 1997). Professional language can help us to mark our territory (Jandt, 2007) and deter service user invaders just as effectively as a high wall can keep intruders out of a private garden. For a reminder of the role that jargon can play in making people vulnerable see Chapter 3. In the next section we will consider some of the ways in which environments in health and social care link to the issues of territoriality explored above.

Territories and Physical Environments

Humans mark territories to denote ownership just as many animals do (although it is difficult to imagine

Space Invaders

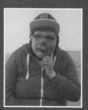

Think about different cultural settings in which you occupy space and consider how you feel and react if others encroach upon your territory in unwanted ways.

Family Lens

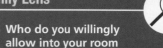

? **Who do you willingly allow into your room at home, and under what circumstances?**

? **How would you feel if a family guest who you didn't know well entered your bedroom for a look round without your permission?**

Social Group Lens

Consider groups that you belong to – this may be a sports or hobby club, or even an online gaming community.

? **How do you react if a stranger who doesn't know the rules of the setting comes and joins you on your home ground and starts to try to get you to behave in line with their rules?**

Professional Lens

? **What spaces do you feel are under your control in the work place?**

? **How may you use language to show that these spaces are controlled by professionals (think of signs, symbols)?**

? **What spaces are controlled by service users?**

Box 6.4: Control of space in different cultural settings a human using lamp posts in quite the same way as dogs do!). We use **boundary markers** such as walls and fences to show the end of one territory and the start of another. The ways in which health and social care buildings are constructed may say something about the values that organisations have as well as marking out the territory. The high walls that were (and sometimes still are) used to separate Victorian era mental institutions from the rest of society were physical examples of the multiple ways in which the inmates were segregated from the rest of society (Goffman, 1968; Goffman, 1961). They stated that they were there to keep the 'abnormal' inmate apart from the rest of 'normal' population. Purpose-built modern health and social care buildings for all types of populations will give consideration not only to the pragmatic ways in which they can promote health and well-being, but also to the overall aesthetic image that says something about the values of the organisation (Verderber, 2010). Bright and light, many buildings suggest efficiency and a desire to create a pleasant environment for interventions (whether they achieve this aim is a matter for debate that goes beyond the bounds of this book). Buildings are therefore not neutral – they are laden with the cultural values of the organisations that construct and occupy them. They will usually be branded with organisational logos (**ear markers** – after the practise of branding cattle (Devito, 1997)) that tell the outside world that this space belongs to the organisation.

Most health and social care staff will not be involved in the design of the buildings that they occupy, but they do have some control over the primary or secondary territories that they inhabit – the work spaces in which they meet service users. Service users will have control over their own homes that staff may visit in their capacity as health and social care workers, but their control over the buildings in which they visit staff is limited. As a health and social care professional, you have the majority of power in determining control of the territory that you inhabit in your work role. The following section will examine how you may control the physical environment and how this links to communication.

CONTROLLING THE PHYSICAL ENVIRONMENT – EFFECTS ON COMMUNICATION

As can be seen from the examples above, territories are linked not only to locations and spaces, but to objects and furnishings that help us to show what those spaces mean to us. These tangible and visible aspects of space make up the physical environment within which we operate. Individuals who are empowered to take charge of a physical space can do so in many ways. They may have control over colour schemes, lighting, temperature, decorations, objects, smells and how furniture is configured (Devito, 1997; Inalhan *et al.*, 2010). All of these factors are linked to communication.

Colour

At the national level of culture , colours have meaning that we take for granted, but that may be understood differently by people from other backgrounds. Even the number of colours that we perceive is influenced by culture. Western cultures may base their words for colour around the colours in the rainbow (seven main colours), but speakers of Bassa base their perceptions around only two (Jandt, 2007). Categorising colours can become very tricky, particularly when they are on the margins of one colour and bordering on the next, and we often have to resort to saying what they are not, to say what they actually are (not blue, not green, but turquoise, for example) (Berger *et al.*, 1969). Having perceived and categorised a colour, we then make unconscious cultural associations to that word or image. For example, whilst white is associated with purity and cleanliness in many Western and Muslim cultures, it is associated with death in Japanese and some Asian cultures (Devito, 1997). White hospital walls could therefore have unintended symbolic meaning when viewed in this context, quite apart from research that suggests that pure white walls can be disorientating and produce extreme behaviours if people are confined within them for long periods (Dalke *et al.*, 2006). Colour perceptions and meanings are therefore not only present at a national level, but also at the level of organisation and professional culture. We are manipulated by colour on a daily basis in all aspects of our lives without necessarily being aware of it. Exposure to different colours can affect our heart rate, respiration and frequency of eye blink, as they have an impact on our emotions (Devito, 1997). Film producers often spend a considerable amount of time considering lighting and colour when creating a product because they know that these factors have an impact at an emotional level that will help to convey the film's message (Kennedy *et al.*, 2002). Some less obvious examples of the link between colour and communication come from the financial sector, which may carefully consider the colour used for a financial report as there is evidence that this may affect the perceptions of investors who are considering the data (Courtis, 2004). Colour, therefore, is perceived to convey meaning to those who are able to see it. Those choosing colour schemes may consciously strive for a particular message to be conveyed, but for those who are the receivers, rather than the creators of the schemes, colour communication generally occurs at a subconscious level

Colour and Communication

Family Lens

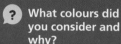

Think about a room that you have had some say in decorating.

(?) What colours did you consider and why?

(?) What colours did you reject and why?

(?) If a stranger were to look at that space, could they guess something about you or your personality from the room?

Professional/Organisational Lens

Have a think about health or social care work spaces that you have visited either as a staff member or a service user.

(?) What colours do health and social care environments tend to go for?

(?) What message do you think this conveys?

Having read the section on colour, have a look at the environment in which you work or go on placement, and think about the communicatively vulnerable clients that may access that environment.

(?) Is there sufficient contrast for those with visual impairment?

(?) Are there too many contrasting colours for those who cannot filter out unwanted stimuli?

(?) If the place is large, are colours used to help direct people who can't read signs?

Box 6.5: Colour and communication under cultural lenses

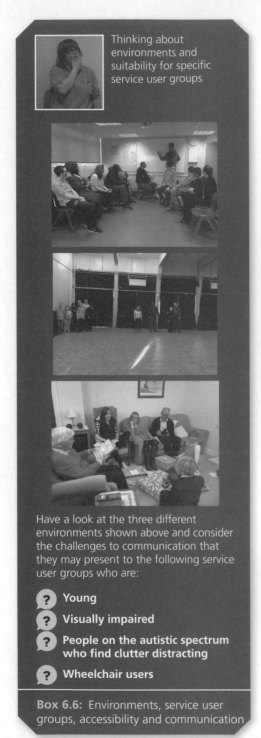

Thinking about environments and suitability for specific service user groups

Have a look at the three different environments shown above and consider the challenges to communication that they may present to the following service user groups who are:

? **Young**

? **Visually impaired**

? **People on the autistic spectrum who find clutter distracting**

? **Wheelchair users**

Box 6.6: Environments, service user groups, accessibility and communication

(Kress, 2009). This subconscious effect is reported to have an impact on the health and well-being, and recovery rates of people in hospital, although definitive empirical research into these effects is limited, possibly because one colour does not suit all. Different client groups may require different types of colour schemes to best meet their needs. For example, those with visual impairment benefit from strongly contrasting colours to differentiate between surfaces, and children may feel more at ease in environments with bright colours (Dalke et al., 2006). However, clients who find it difficult to filter out stimuli such as those on the autistic spectrum, with dementia or learning disability may find too many bright colours distracting (Dijkstra et al., 2008). They may, however, benefit from colour-coded environments to help them find their way around new places (Dalke et al., 2006). Colours for different floors on a hospital or different departments can help (provided the common colours associated with colour blindness such as blue and green are avoided). Have a go at the exercise in Box 6.5 to explore how colour and meaning may be linked in your own life. Whilst you may not select the colours for the environments within which you have face to face interactions with service users, it is important to consider that these may have a much stronger influence on vulnerable communicators than you may imagine. Colour is not limited to the physical environment – it is also present in the colours you wear. White clothing in a hospital environment is often associated with dominance, and many other dominant disciplines such as solicitors and police are associated with black clothing (Vrij et al., 2005). Patterned clothing may be distracting (Dijkstra et al., 2008). People who are distracted by what you wear will not be concentrating on what you wish to communicate, and if you wish to empower people then you need to present a non-dominant image from the outset. If you have the opportunity to select your own clothing or influence the choice of colours of uniform, then it is worth bearing in mind that single, pastel colours may facilitate communication with those who are communicatively vulnerable. Clothing will be considered in more depth in the next chapter of this book when we consider the performance that health and social care staff put on for service users when they interact together.

Lighting

Lighting and colour are strongly linked, as colours reflect different amounts of light. The best colour scheme will not be effective if the lighting is poor. Good quality lighting can affect both mood and communication. Not only can poor lighting make it harder for people to navigate (particularly if they have visual impairment), it can also make it harder for those with hearing loss to lip read (Dalke *et al.*, 2006; Lieu *et al.*, 2007) and make people feel depressed (Dalke *et al.*, 2006). All these factors can impact upon communication, and well-lit environments are more likely to facilitate communication with people who are vulnerable because of mental health problems or sensory impairment. However, not all light is good light. Lighting that is too bright, or that creates glare, can be difficult for people with visual impairment (Cook *et al.*, 2005), and this can become particularly important with people who also have hearing loss who need to lip read (such as many elderly individuals). Fluorescent lighting flickers around 60 times every second. For most people, this is unnoticable, but for those who are particularly sensitive to sensory stimuli (such as those on the autistic spectrum), this can be very distracting and distressing (Colman *et al.*, 1976; O'Leary *et al.*, 1978). A well-lit room with diffused, incandescent or natural illumination can create an environment that supports communication for most service users, and rooms with dimmer lights that can vary the illumination to meet particular visual needs are ideal.

Health and social care staff need to remember that although the service user may know what type of lighting suits them best, they are unlikely to volunteer this information unless specifically asked since staff control this territory. They may, however, communicate their discomfort through their body language or apparent lack of concentration. Asking people who appear uncomfortable about whether there is anything in the environment that can be altered to make it easier to communicate can be an important question for staff to have in their repertoire. People who do not use words to communicate may be reacting to the lights that are distracting them – you may not sense this, but they do, and if you don't address this, the lights will have a greater say in the exchange than you do.

An Ordinary Ward Round?

Communicate2U members can be highly sensitive to sensory stimuli that others may not notice.

They have created a film to show you how this may affect them whilst they are interacting with you.

Although the film is set in a hospital, the factors apply in any setting where staff meet service users.

The film is humorous but the underlying message is serious: if you don't attend to the sensory input in the environment, we won't be focusing on what you want us to hear!

You can see this film on the website. Whilst watching it think about the following:

? **What sensory input do Communicate2U members find hard to cope with?**

? **How does this impact upon the communication exchange?**

? **How much of a role does the service user play in the interaction?**

? **What small things could the staff do to improve the environment to make it less distracting?**

Box 6.7: An ordinary ward round? The impact of the senses on communication

Temperature

The temperature at which people feel comfortable can vary widely between individuals, and those who are very young, old or unwell may have different thermal comfort requirements to staff (Lomas *et al.*, 2012). If people are too warm or too cold this can affect their ability to concentrate during an interaction. The dominant person within an environment generally has more opportunity to influence the ambient temperature (Inalhan *et al.*, 2010). If a member of health or social care staff is doing a visit to a service user's home and the temperature is uncomfortable for them, but right for the service user, this may make it harder for the professional. However, it may also communicate to them that some of the client's basic needs are being considered. It may be difficult for staff to alter the temperature in their professional environment to meet the needs of each person that enters, but some basic consideration of the ambient temperature that is likely to be most supportive for the majority of clients seen may facilitate communication. Noting body language that may indicate that someone is too hot or cold and either offering to make an adjustment or apologising for the lack of temperature control communicates concern, even if nothing practical can be done.

Olfactics – The Science of Smell

Anybody who thinks that smell can't communicate a message may like to consider the many millions of pounds that are spent upon advertising and buying perfumes and aftershaves each year. The science of smell – **olfactics** – is big business. Smell is a primeval sense that has a very close link to our emotions and memory since information from the cells that detect smell is sent both to the olfactory bulb of the brain and the limbic system, which helps to regulate emotions. Infants recognise their mothers partly according to the smell of their milk (Gazzaniga *et al.*, 2002) and this sense does not require high levels of cognition to provoke an emotional response. We all have individual scents, and in some Arab countries, an acceptable personal distance for communication is one that allows participants to smell one another's breath (Jandt, 2007). The types of messages associated with personal odour are attraction messages, memory messages and identification messages (Devito, 1997). Whether the original smell that a person has is acceptable or not is culturally determined – people in Western cultures often spend a significant amount of time and effort masking this smell in a way that people in Arab cultures may find puzzling or devious (Jandt, 2007).

The environments in which health and social care staff work are going to smell. To what degree and what they smell of will vary, but each time we perceive a scent, however unconsciously, we will pick up a message. Staff who enter a service user's home may make a decision about the cleanliness and lifestyle of the person based upon the smell of the person, and that judgement will most likely be culturally grounded (Dana, 2011). For example, a city-dwelling professional who does a home visit to a farm may well feel some discomfort at the smell of manure that pervades the home and may then unconsciously be more alert for signs of dirt when doing the visit. Similarly, service users and carers who enter health and social care environments will pick up on the smell and make a judgement about the organisation or professional that has created it. The smell

Objects and Meaning

 Have a look at the picture below and think about what that object means to you:

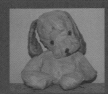

Most people seeing that picture will not have a strong emotional reaction; it may communicate that this is a toy that was loved and is cute (or ugly depending upon your preference), maybe something that is meant for children. Possibly dirty and ready for the scrap heap. Members of cultures that have no history of teddy bears may view it perhaps as a hunter's talisman. However, for the original owner of the teddy it holds a wealth of meaning; a symbol of security during childhood, a link to a happy era and a precious object that could never be replaced by a replica or substitute.

Have a think about an object that you own that you love and cherish.

? **What does the object mean to you?**

? **Why?**

? **How may other people who have no knowledge of you view it?**

? **How would you feel if someone touched it without your express permission?**

Now look at another object that can have a lot of meaning for service users who own one: a wheelchair.

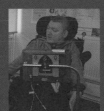

? **What meaning does a wheelchair convey to you?**

Objects as markers

Think about how you may feel in the following situations:

• Somebody comes into your bedroom and tidies it without your prior knowledge or permission

• You go to the swimming pool on holiday and all of the deckchairs are covered in towels, yet the majority are not occupied

• How would you react if you then met the person who had tidied the room, or put the towel on the chair for 3 hours before coming to sit on it?

Box 6.8: Objects and meaning

of disinfectant, for example, may not be one that people would normally rate as positive, but in a hospital setting it can give a sense of reassurance that the environment is clean (Baccarani et al., 2014). Conversely, it may trigger off unpleasant memories of previous painful or embarrassing encounters for service users who may then become anxious. Staff who work in these environments become culturally blind to the smells of their work place and may not notice the multitude of odours. Odours may include the smell of bodies and the cleaning fluids used to mask or neutralise them. Although they are familiar and unnoticeable to staff, many service users will notice and respond to the message that the smell is sending to them.

It may not be possible to control the smells in an environment (although steps may be taken to minimise these). However, health and social care staff need to be very mindful of the cultural nature of smell messages before making judgements about others, and before labelling a service user's behaviour as disruptive. There are a multitude of reasons as to why someone may smell the way that they do. A seemingly aggressive service user may be scared by the smell of the place that reminds them of their last horrible experience in a health or social care setting. An unpleasant smell (such as urine) in a service user's home may send a powerful message that someone is not coping and may need additional support or monitoring. Vulnerable service users may be living in situations in which those that care for them try to mask issues that are areas of legitimate concern for staff. Someone who is reliant upon carers for washing and dressing and who smells of urine and faeces on multiple occasions may be a service user who is at risk. As long as there is some sensitivity in how that message is explored and interpreted, smell within an environment may send a message for help that a communicatively vulnerable service user is otherwise unable to articulate.

Objects

Objects within an environment can communicate meaning. They can be used to indicate who is dominant in a particular space, for example. **Central markers** are objects that are used to lay claim to a territory (e.g. placing a towel over a deck chair); **boundary markers** show where one territory ends and another starts (e.g. a filing cabinet that separates one desk area from another), and **earmarkers** denote affiliation to a particular group (e.g. clothing with a logo on it to denote which organisation a person belongs to). On paper, the use of objects to mark territory may sound quite unemotive, but many people get quite defensive and upset if someone removes a towel from a deckchair, for example. Humans like to defend their spaces and can feel threatened when markers are not respected. Health and social care staff will often enter service user's spaces where such markers are present. In the hospital setting, the curtains around the bed denote boundaries, and clients will usually have placed objects on lockers. Staff will be used to those spaces being occupied on a temporary basis, and will have routines for maintaining them that they know must be adhered to. At some level, whether consciously or unconsciously, they will consider it to be their territory (Weeks et al., 1979). As such they may enter it with limited formality, moving objects as needed to maintain standards of hygiene that are the norm for that organisational culture. For service users, however, the space that has become their secondary territory can become very personal, and markers being moved may feel threatening or disrespectful (Woogara, 2005). For some communicatively vulnerable people (such as those on the autistic spectrum) having particular objects in particular places can be a very important part of feeling safe in a strange and threatening environment, and having objects moved can be distressing. Similar situations can occur when staff visit service users in their own environments. For example, grandpa's chair may be marked by his jumper, and everyone (except the unsuspecting member of staff who is visiting) knows not to sit in it. Staff who are respectful of what the position of objects may mean to service users who are already under stress are communicating that they recognise the importance of having a place to feel safe in. Asking permission (verbally or non-verbally) before moving something in a service user's space communicates to that person that you know that this space is important to them, they are worthy of the kind of respect that you yourself would like to have shown to you. Have a go at the exercise in Box 6.8 to explore how you may react if your possessions are not respected.

The meaning that objects hold is constructed at both a personal and cultural level. Take the example of a chair – it's obvious that it's something to sit on, isn't it? In fact, we only know it is something to sit on because that is knowledge that has been culturally agreed. In many cultures the natural way to rest when not standing is to squat, and even in the Western world chairs only started to be commonly used from the sixteenth century (Ingold, 2004). Chairs may have other meanings in different

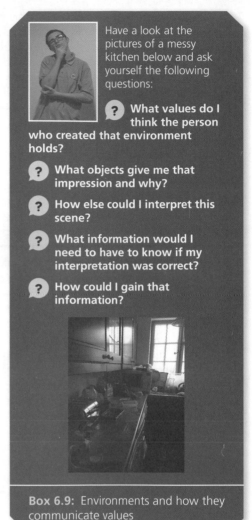

Have a look at the pictures of a messy kitchen below and ask yourself the following questions:

? **What values do I think the person who created that environment holds?**

? **What objects give me that impression and why?**

? **How else could I interpret this scene?**

? **What information would I need to have to know if my interpretation was correct?**

? **How could I gain that information?**

Box 6.9: Environments and how they communicate values

cultural groups. For people who use a wheelchair, the chair may be considered as an extension of their own body (Iwakuma, 2002), and health or social care staff who touch the chair without permission may be considered to have entered into intimate space in a threatening and insulting way. Cultural differences in how objects are used abound. I learned this as a newly qualified therapist doing a home visit with a family newly arrived in the UK. My confusion as to why a relatively agile grandfather was reported to be having difficulties managing to use the toilet was lifted when I observed him trying to climb onto the toilet seat and balance on the rim around the hole. His previous experience of relieving himself was squatting over a hole in the ground. We had different cultural assumptions relating to toileting, and my suggestion that he sit to use the facility was met with some disgust.

I privately thought that his actions were primitive; he thought my suggestions were unhygienic and odd. Both of us made negative cultural judgements about the other and the issue of toileting remained unresolved. We also assumed similarity of customs instead of difference, which is a barrier to cultural understanding (Barna, 1997). The exercises in Boxes 6.8 and 6.9 explore how cultural meanings may be attached to objects and their use within specific environments.

The above examples introduce the idea that objects such as furniture speak to us in cultural ways. The ways in which furniture in environments is configured not only supports or hinders interpersonal communication, but also communicates something about the power relationship between participants in an interaction (Davis, 1984; Seabury, 1971). An individual seated behind an object such as a desk or a clip board is symbolising their relative authority and potential dominance even before they have opened their mouth to speak. In their work place, health and social care staff may take pains to try to eliminate these physical barriers to communication. However, the space in which the communication takes place will indicate something about the position in the hierarchy that the person occupies and the values that they hold. Professional text books on book shelves may say something about how keen the member of staff is to keep up to date with current practice (are the books dusty). The arrangement of chairs may indicate how carefully the member of staff has considered the need to facilitate communication (and therefore what value that holds for them). Staff who visit service users in their homes will evaluate information from the environment to help them make judgements about the person, and this may happen as a conscious part of a formal assessment or be an unconscious process. Service users who live in a house that is untidy, visibly dirty, with no books may be judged differently to ones who live in homes that are spotless and filled with diplomas and reading material (Devito, 1997). Environments are only part of the story – the person occupying the book-filled office may never read the texts; the untidy, dirty house may be filled with a close-knit family of animal lovers who are rarely home and the spotless home may house a family which gives an outward appearance of respectability but hides domestic violence. They do, however, often communicate the values that people hold, or wish to portray to others. Watzlawick (1978; 2010) argues that humans and their environment are interrelated and that to understand communication, the physical context in which it occurs has to be considered. The scenario in Box 6.10 illustrates this point:

Imran's Door and Communication

Imran is sitting at home watching the cricket on TV when he hears the front door slam loudly. He hurriedly reaches for the remote and switches over to a history channel, shoving the packet of biscuits down the side of the sofa as he does so. His wife comes into the room with a scowl on her face and he glances up expectantly, trying to look innocent.

Box 6.10: Environments and how they communicate with us: Imran's example

In this case, the object that communicates meaning and changes Imran's behaviour is the slamming door. Imran has heard that type of door slam before and knows that his wife is in a bad mood as she returns home from work. She disapproves of the amount of time he spends watching sport and wants him to improve his mind. She has also commented upon his increase in weight. The door slam symbolises an unpleasant evening that he wishes to avoid, and the TV channel and biscuits symbolise his straying from her stated values. You are reminded of Malcolm's use of biscuits as an object to take power within a social care setting that was used within Chapter 2 (Malcom's quotation). He understood that the act of providing a drink fulfilled a cultural convention that helped families to feel more comfortable in situations that were otherwise dominated by social care staff. His ploy of presenting a packet of biscuits communicated his desire for drinks to be provided without him explicitly having to make a request that could have been refused. Chapter 2 explicitly argued that knowledge equates to power, and knowledge of cultural conventions and the objects that are linked to them can be a powerful tool in the communication toolbox of health and social care staff too; especially if they have to face Malcolm wielding a packet of rich tea biscuits!

Many of the objects that health and social care staff use or have in their environments will hold symbolic meaning for themselves and service users, but the meaning may be different for each cultural group. Taking the example of the clipboard again, for the member of staff it may be a useful tool for information gathering that has little emotional meaning. For the service user or family member it may be one more symbol of their lives being dissected by a stranger who will be adding to the already thick case folder and it may be an unwelcome symbol of intrusion. During an initial encounter, service users may well be reacting to the symbol, rather than the person behind it. Staff who have an awareness of how objects communicate may be more understanding and able to work through initial difficulties in such situations.

Familiarity of Environment and Emotional Communication

National Lens

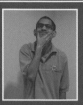

Imagine that you are in an unfamiliar country on holiday and you have gone to a marketplace with your family. The buildings, trees and objects all look strange and you are surrounded by odd smells and loud noises that make no sense to you. Suddenly you realise that the people that were with you have vanished. You are alone. You start to look around for someone to help you and a stranger grabs your arm and starts to lead you away from where your family was.

? **How do you feel?**

? **How do you react?**

Service users in an unfamiliar setting may feel exactly the same way if they are unable to understand or recall what is happening to them.

? **How may service users feel in a strange environment if a strange member of staff starts to take them somewhere new?**

? **How may they react?**

? **How could you give them some reassurance without using words? (Think of the power of familiar objects)**

Box 6.11: Unfamiliar environments and emotional communication

Bringing it All Together – Sensory Integration

As you may have gathered, this chapter illustrates how everything around us communicates something. Our senses are assaulted by noises, smells, colours and shapes and different forms of touch (such as temperature). In familiar situations this constant bombardment is not noticed by the majority of people as they automatically filter out unnecessary stimuli to focus on what they deem to be important. Viewers intent on a basketball game can fail to see a person in a gorilla suit who invades a pitch (Simons *et al.*, 1999), so you can imagine how easily we can filter out the mundane. This filtering helps us to cope in a world that would otherwise constantly be shouting out messages to us. However, a significant number of people have difficulty in processing and filtering sensory information. People on the autistic spectrum (Jones *et al.*, 2003; Tomchek *et al.*, 2007), people with a learning disability (Ayres, 1979; Schaaf *et al.*, 2005), schizophrenia (Leitman *et al.*, 2005) and dementia (Livingston *et al.*, 2014) are amongst the populations that have been identified as having additional difficulties with sensory processing. These are the types of populations that have

---

Communicating your Values through the Environment

Family Cultural Lens

Have a look around a room in your home and examine all the ways in which the room communicates the values that your family hold

Professional and Cultural Lens

Think about a professional workspace which you have worked in or visited.

Consider all the things that we have covered in this chapter:

? **Who chooses how the territory looks?**

? **Size of the space?**

? **How it looks?**

- Type of lighting
- Colours and contrasts
- Objects
- Types and position of furniture

? **How it smells?**

? **How it sounds?**

? **The texture of objects and furnishings?**

Imagine you are a service user entering the place for the first time.

? **What does this environment say to you about the values of the professionals that work there?**

? **If you found new smells and noises difficult to cope with, how challenging would that room be?**

If you were in charge of redesigning the room to make it a safe environment for people who are communicatively vulnerable to meet in what would you do?

If you were the professional using that room before the redesign, what small changes could you make to help people who are vulnerable?

Box 6.12: Recognising power within the environment and reducing the effects of staff domination

been identified throughout this book as being communicatively vulnerable. The exercise in Box 6.11 is designed to help you understand how someone with communication difficulties and sensory processing problems may experience a new setting such as a hospital or social care environment. These physical environments can be awash with new sensory experiences that can make them very frightening places, even for people who don't have additional communication needs (Baccarani *et al.*, 2014). For someone who cannot understand where they are, why the familiar sights, sounds, smells and people have disappeared, it can be terrifying, and they are unable to express this fear in words. They may do so by presenting with behaviours that staff then label as challenging.

The use of sensory stimuli to help us to modify how we feel is something that is familiar to most people. We may seek comfort from a hug, a bottle of wine, a bar of chocolate (or all three) if we are feeling down. On a long car journey we may open a window or turn the radio up to help keep ourselves awake and focused. People who have difficulties with sensory integration may also use these types of strategies to help themselves stay calm (Tomchek *et al.*, 2007), but their techniques may look unusual to staff who are not familiar with sensory approaches to behaviour. They may need specific sensory items to be near them, or may rock to provide themselves with sensory input that is otherwise absent. If the environment is shouting out that it is scary and threatening, these objects become even more important. Familiar sensory items can communicate a sense of safety and security. People may need to feel particular textured objects, have some smells that they are very sensitive to eliminated or reduced, or have environments in which unfamiliar noises can be minimised. Health and social care staff who ask service users or carers what objects or actions help a person to feel safe are achieving two key communication goals. They are moderating the information that the scary environment is sending and they are communicating to those individuals that they understand they may have additional needs and wish to help. Both these messages are likely to improve the communication between staff and communicatively vulnerable people. You may not be able to make large changes to the environments in which you work, but you can certainly make small changes that have the potential to make a big difference to vulnerable people. Just recognising the need to do so gives a very powerful message: you are important to me and I care enough to try to make you more comfortable. Have a go at the exercise in Box 6.12 to get an idea of the power that the environment (and you) holds, and what you could do to redress the balance of power with vulnerable service users.

CHAPTER SUMMARY

Health and social care staff often have spaces that they control in which they interact with service users. These territories tend to fade into the background and become invisible to professionals, but for the service users that enter them they are new environments that send a wealth of information about the person that they are communicating with and the organisation in which they work. Staff who make a conscious effort to attend to the messages that the physical environment sends out to people can improve the chances of effective communication. They have the power to either attend to environmental messages or to ignore them, but by doing the latter they are running the risk of creating spaces in which communicatively vulnerable people are oppressed or disadvantaged in a communication exchange.

EASY READ CHAPTER SUMMARY

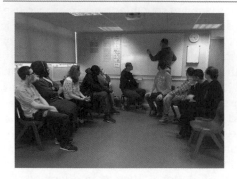

The way a room looks can make us feel good or bad

It can also make it easier or harder for people to communicate

The room in the picture is a classroom

It is not too busy. That makes it easier to listen and learn

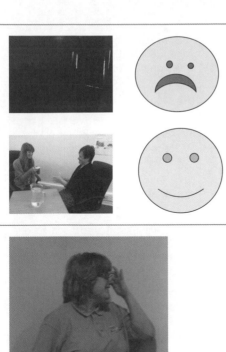

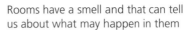

Dark rooms where it is hard to see can make us feel bad

Brighter rooms can make us feel good if the light is right

Neon lights can make it hard for some people to think

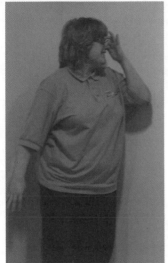

Pooh! Horrible cheese smell!

Rooms have a smell and that can tell us about what may happen in them

A smell may remind us of good or bad things that have happened before

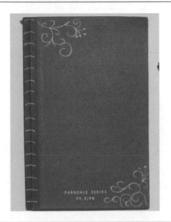

Objects in rooms also tell us about the people that live there

Some people who find it hard to cope in hospitals may need special things to hold to help them stay calm

This may be something they have at home – like a special book with pictures of family in it

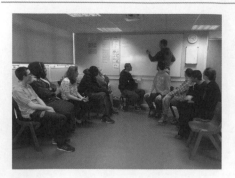

If staff make rooms look good and friendly, it makes it easier for everyone to communicate

This room doesn't look too busy

It has some simple pictures on the walls to help people understand what will happen

The room isn't smelly, and it is bright

It has a light switch so if someone finds it too bright it can be made darker

The chairs are comfortable. People are allowed to move them to a place that feels right

PERFORMING INCLUSIVE HEALTH AND SOCIAL CARE SCRIPTS

Aims

By the end of this chapter you will be able to:

➡ Understand the concept of performance scripts

➡ Identify the components that make up the script of your own profession

➡ Compare the performance scripts of professionals in health and social care with those of vulnerable communicators

➡ Analyse how your own professional script could be altered to be culturally sensitive to the needs of communicatively vulnerable people.

INTRODUCTION

Whether we are conscious of it or not, nearly all of us are actors that consummately play a wide range of different roles throughout our lives. We may be sons or daughters, siblings, parents, friends, students, teachers or health and social care professionals. Each time we slip into one of these roles, we behave and communicate differently to fit into the cultural norms that are associated with that title. Even in the same role, our act may change as soon as we encounter a different audience. Unless the situation is new or difficult we usually don't even think about how we go about those roles – we just act and react. The exercise in Box 7.1 illustrates how we may do this within the family setting.

The exercises throughout this book have been designed to help you understand the different ways that you communicate and behave in the different cultural groups to which you belong. By now you should be aware that the types of body language that you use, the words and phrases that you select and the power that you have to structure the environment varies in different cultural settings. You should also be aware that no matter how low down in the hierarchy you may think you are at work, in comparison to the vast majority of service users, you are powerful. You know the language, the systems and set the format for interactions. Most of this occurs without your conscious

Performing Life – Family Lens

Think of a time when your family has been expecting guests – for example, for a visit or for a party.

? **How did the house look before the visit?**

? **How did family members interact with one another whilst preparations were underway?**

? **How did family members interact once guests arrived?**

? **How did family members interact with one another once the guests departed?**

If the house looked the same and family interactions in front of guests were performed in the same way as in private, then you are part of a very small minority of people indeed who are happy to present no alternative face to the outside world.

Within the Western world, our roles as family members are usually performed in a less formal manner. We usually change the performance to a more formal one in front of guests.

Box 7.1: Changing the act for different audiences

awareness as you are a part of the culture. If you have read through the chapters in this book and taken part in the exercises, that previously hidden knowledge should now be something of which you have conscious awareness. This final chapter aims to help you to use that awareness to prepare a professional script that includes all communicatively vulnerable people. It will not require you to learn a different way of working for each labelled condition, but instead will explore some basic principles of communication that cross cultural boundaries. It will ask you to apply what you do quite naturally in other cultural settings to your professional role. It therefore isn't hard – but it can help to reduce the risk of already vulnerable people being further marginalised and put at risk by the very people whose job it is to support them.

PERFORMING LIFE AND EXCLUDING VULNERABLE PEOPLE

Life is complex, but by comparing it to a play it is possible to look at some of the components that make up everyday interactions. This can help us to try to understand not only how they play out now, but also how they could work better in the future. Goffman is an author whose work in this area has been very influential. His ideas have many links with the concept of face (presenting ourselves in a good light in front of others (Goffman, 1967; Goffman, 1959)), which is also a big part of intercultural theory (Jandt, 2007). Goffman's theories have been used elsewhere to describe how professionals in health and social care act to present themselves to their service user and carer audience in a manner that is consistent with stated organisational values (Goffman, 1968; Goffman, 1963; John, 1996). These studies, however, have not considered in depth what happens if one of the parties present has no ability to change their performance because they lack the cognitive ability to do so. Some people with a severe learning disability or mental health need may fall into this category and are particularly vulnerable if their scripted ways of behaving don't fit with the performance that staff expect of them, and staff are unable to change their own performance. This section will look at the elements that make up performances such as setting, appearance, manner and scripts to help to explore how professionals and communicatively vulnerable service users and their carers may act when they come together.

In Chapter 1 you were introduced to the concept of high and low context cultures. Low context cultures rely on words to communicate the message and health and social care cultures were identified as tending towards this style. In high context cultures, each person knows a lot about the values and communication style of the other person, and they have a pre-set script that helps them to know how to communicate and behave without them having to use a lot of words (Jandt, 2007; Scollon *et al.*, 2012). Communicatively vulnerable people and support workers interacting well together often adopt this cultural style. When people with similar cultural styles of communication meet there are usually few problems – they all know what performance is expected and things go smoothly. However, problems occur when people from low and high context cultures meet. Each expects the other to interact in the way that they are familiar with. When this doesn't happen the result is confusion, disharmony and an assumption that the other person is acting in a deliberately rude or obstructive way. The key to improving communication is for at least one of those present to recognise that the problem may be due to a difference in cultural styles of communicating. That person can then try to adapt their own performance so that it is closer in style to the other individual (Barna, 1997; Jandt, 2007; Neuliep, 2009; Scollon *et al.*, 2012). As noted above, many vulnerable people will not have the ability to change their script; the onus is therefore upon you, the professional, to take responsibility for altering your performance when this type of culture clash happens in the health or social care setting.

The concept of how professional roles should be acted exists even before students start to study (Horsburgh *et al.*, 2006). When you selected your career, it is very unlikely that you did so at random: you will have had knowledge as to how your professional role is generally acted (whether that was gained by real-life observations, discussions, TV or by reading about it). Most people will then have decided they could imagine themselves acting that role in the future, and prepared themselves for the role before filling in application forms and going for interviews. They then learn about the role in a technical way once they enter formal education (see Chapter 1 if you need to refresh your memory on how culture is learned). The role of the vulnerable service user is one that is informally shaped by the dominant members of society, and is not one that people select for themselves. If dominant members of society values things such as the ability to be fluent with words, to be critical and reflective, and humanity is defined according to these terms (Friere, 1986), then people who can't achieve this are inadvertently defined as less than human. This creates very real problems for the people who are implicitly put into this non-human category since they are then excluded from the moral rights that are accorded to the rest of the population. However, the rest of the population may not even be consciously aware of behaving in this way. It can be hard to change cultural knowledge that has been learned informally, but altering taught technical knowledge can promote more rapid cultural change (Hall, 1959). Therefore, the way in which health and social care students are educated about vulnerable service users is a potentially valuable tool for cultural change in health and social care. However, this can only happen if the values and communication styles of the marginalised cultural group inform and underpin education strategies.

Health and social care students and professionals are a part of a culture that values the principles of critical reflection advocated by Friere (1986). They have roles in which it is important to show a good professional front (Goffman, 1959). They are also members of a wider culture that has often removed people who find words hard (such as those with a learning disability) from society for generations (Atkinson *et al.*, 2000; Goodey, 2004; Nind *et al.*, 2010; Potts, 2000). Cultures have historically used segregation as a means of dealing with people who do not fit with cultural norms (Berger *et al.*, 1969). The result of this segregation is that members of the dominant culture have no effective scripts to fall back on when faced with people whose values and communication styles fall outside of their experience. If you haven't had experience of communicating effectively with people who don't use words to communicate, you may be fearful, not know what to do, or may not even try to communicate, as the quotation from Trudy illustrates:

Trudy:	*... unfortunately, I think that some people ... will never open their eyes to that* (seeing a person with a learning disability as a person who communicates).
Annette:	*What do you think stops them opening their eyes?*
Trudy:	*Maybe lack of education, probably lack of education. ... I think for a lot of people, unless you have come into contact with it ... whether it's a family member, you know ... you never have to deal with it really. And it's only until you start having to deal with it that you realise that* [they can communicate in their own way] *... people can be forgotten.*

Communicate2U quotation 7.1: Trudy explains how people learn to communicate with those who are vulnerable

When we are faced with people who seem different, the natural tendency is to label them as 'the other' and to define them by what they are not (Shome, 1996). Labelling a person who does not use words well as being a poor communicator or as non-communicative gives people who use words well the excuse to not try to communicate with them. They are not fully human and so are not accorded with the values and support that would be offered to a more articulate service user. This interpretation could explain why vulnerable people who could not speak were overlooked in hospitals (Francis, 2013), were not offered basic investigations that could have prevented unnecessary deaths (Heslop *et al.*, 2013; Mencap, 2013; Mencap, 2006; Michael *et al.*, 2008) or were supported in social care in ways that denied them their basic human rights (DoH, 2012; Flynn *et al.*, 2013). However, performances can change, and the sections below are designed to help you to think about how you could change how you act so that you avoid similar events from occurring when you work in health and social care environments.

HEALTH AND SOCIAL CARE PERFORMANCE SCRIPTS

Scripts are part of the traditions that are embedded within cultures, but fortunately for us, we only have to learn a relatively small number of performances to be effective, since many scripts are transferrable (Goffman, 1967; Goffman, 1959). For example, you will have a script to deal with people who are strangers to you or known to you. In new situations you will start off a meeting with one of those basic scripts that you then adapt as you go along. Health and social care professionals have particular scripts to help guide their performances (Goffman, 1968; Goffman, 1967; Goffman, 1961; Goffman, 1959). Performance scripts include the following components:

- The role and the degree to which the player believes in the performance
- The personal setting – appearance and manner adopted in front of others
- The objects used during the performance
- The activities and routines that make up the performance
- The script followed
- The physical setting – the environment

The physical setting was the focus of Chapter 6 – the rest of this chapter will focus upon your own personal performance.

ROLE AND ROLE SINCERITY

Before starting this section, have a go at the exercise in Box 7.2 and be very honest with yourself about the reasons you had for selecting your profession, and how you feel now that you have had some training or experience. When you went for your interview to get into your professional training, you were probably asked why you wanted to

Role Sincerity – Professional Lens

Be totally honest with yourself and (in order of priority) list the top 5 reasons why you chose your profession or current post:

1.
2.
3.
4.
5.

Now compare this to the values that your profession has listed as priorities.

Have a look at the spectrum shown below and rate, on an average day, how sincerely you believe in your professional values.

Very sincere ...	Cynical
(Fully believe ...	Don't think they reflect the reality I work in)

Now think about what factors have influenced where you are on the spectrum and list:

Things I could personally change to move closer to values	Things I can't personally change to move closer to values

Box 7.2: Professional role sincerity and cynicism

do the course. Have a look at the questions in Box 7.3 to see some potential responses to that question:

	Question	Response
A	Why do you want to do this training?	'I will be trained to get a job that earns me a reasonable wage, that has good chances for job security, and that I think will interest me.'
B	Why do you want to do this training?	'I'm caring, I want to make a difference and help people. This job does that.'

Box 7.3: Role sincerity in the interview process

It's very unlikely that successful candidates into the profession answered with A. However, for some people, the first response may be the more truthful one at the start of training, and for some, the second; for most people, if they are very honest, it is probably a mixture of both. The National Health Service in the UK is currently committed to values-based recruitment (NHS, 2015b) and asks employers and educators to examine applicants on the basis of their values in order to address some of the health inequalities that have emerged in the reports into ill treatment of vulnerable people referenced above. This is, however, complex for a number of reasons. People may fully and sincerely believe in the values of the role that they embody, or they may be quite cynical about the values that are espoused, but can hide this (Goffman, 1959). They may enter a role in a cynical frame of mind, yet end up fully believing as training helps them to understand their profession. Alternatively, they may become more cynical as they play the role and it fails to live up to the values they thought they had signed up to (Goffman, 1968; Goffman, 1967; Goffman, 1961; Goffman, 1959). This book has argued that if professionals truly wish to live up to the standards of caring that are the foundation of health and social care roles, then they need to do so in such a way as to make basic communication with the most communicatively vulnerable a core component of everybody's repertoire. For this to occur there needs to be a cultural shift towards sincere and meaningful engagement with *all* service users throughout the professional journey, not just the ones who are articulate and easy to engage with. The starting point for cultural change is often the next generation who can adopt new ideas and transmit them through existing cultures (Jandt, 2007). The starting point for the professional journey is the recruitment and training process.

Training experiences clearly play an important role in how sincerely people believe in their profession (Goffman, 1959), and because training of professionals is explicit and technical (Chapter 1), it is the easiest way to effect cultural change (Hall, 1959). However, since professionals that provide training are often members of the cultures that have not supported communicatively vulnerable service users well, there is a danger that the patterns of ineffective communication will be replicated in future generations as this is usually how cultural knowledge is transmitted (Berger *et al.*, 1969). There is therefore an argument that *in order to be culturally competent, health and social care professionals need to learn how to communicate by learning from those people who are communicatively vulnerable*. This gives a rationale for the need for service user involvement that is a requirement of many UK courses, and would require students to actually experience communication with people who find words difficult. Currently, whilst UK course requirements often include the need for service user involvement, there is no set requirement, or agreement as to how this should occur (for examples see COT, 2015; Hill *et al.*, 2014; Narey, 2014). Historically, there have been a wide range of degrees of service user involvement in professional training: from one-off, tokenistic sessions, to actors playing the part of people with disabilities, through to service users being fully engaged in the design and delivery of programmes (Towle *et al.*, 2010). This book argues that all professionals should have training from people who are communicatively vulnerable, and that those people delivering the training should be seen as experts in their own communication styles. This presents many ethical challenges to organisations that may have limited experience in adapting their communication to include people who find words hard. As members of the disempowering cultures, they are unlikely to see that they have difficulties with their communication and are therefore likely to be ineffective when it comes to exploring effective support mechanisms to create a safe and welcoming environment for vulnerable people. However, there are numerous organisations that sit outside of universities or health and social care organisations that have expertise in working in partnership with vulnerable service users. Creating partnerships with such organisations can be beneficial for both parties if each recognises the cultural expertise of the other.

The experiences of professionals and students who have been taught by members of Communicate2U illustrate that adopting an intercultural approach to learning can be a quick and effective method for improving communication between professionals and vulnerable communicators. Teaching sessions are based on the premise that as professionals normally have the power within communication exchanges, they need to experience the disempowerment that comes from having to use a form of communication with which they are less familiar. People with a learning disability, mental health issues, sensory impairment and significant physical health needs that require the use of a voice communication aid lead the sessions. They are presented as cultural communication experts and use a range of creative media (such as drama, music or art, which are less word-based) to teach the students. Most students are initially very uncomfortable with this reversal of roles. They feel disempowered as they don't know what to expect and aren't familiar with the communication form. Research into these experiences suggests that this type of face to face interaction with people who they would normally view as having communication deficits had more impact and veracity than a word based lecture on communication skills delivered by a health or social care professional as the quotations overleaf illustrate:

Some of the students had previously experienced role play scenarios with people who acted the part of vulnerable communicators. Despite this, until they actually interacted with this client group, they lacked confidence in their communication skills. They noted that there was no substitute for real interactions with people who were members of the culture that communicates in different ways:

Student 1:   *Actually having to communicate with the person made you think about a lot more things than a lecture or seminar would ... it was really effective.*

Student2:   *I think if it was done without the examples it would almost be kind of you'd walk out the lecture hall and not really remember it because the people there have got a much bigger impact on what we think and what we can think about on placement and practice.*

Communicate2U quotation 7.2: Students' experiences of intercultural learning

Expert Trainers under the Cultural Lens

Think about the following:

? **How much training does your professional programme provide to ensure that you are comfortable communicating with people who find words hard?**

? **Who provides that training? (e.g. staff or service users/carers)**

? **How do you learn (lecture, video, face to face)?**

? **How well does the training link to professional values of inclusion for the most vulnerable communicators?**

? **If your training doesn't include training from people from the cultures in which words are not the primary form of communication, why do you think this happens?**

? **How will you address that gap?**

Box 7.4: Who trains you in communication skills? Training under the cultural lens

If health and social care professionals are sincere in their stated values of not marginalising the most vulnerable communicators, then serious consideration has to be given as to how to give them a valued role as a cultural communication expert within training programmes. Many people with different communication strengths struggle to find employment, despite being keen to be in a work role. Some may wish to undertake a teaching role within health and social care programmes if this is an option. Provided that careful consideration is given to how communicatively vulnerable people are supported throughout the process of engaging with organisations that are culturally biased towards the use of words, this can be a valuable experience for service users and students alike (Thomas *et al.*, 2014). However, such programmes are not the norm, and some health and social care students may only engage with service users who are articulate or with actors playing the role of people who find words hard. In the UK during the 1970s, a popular TV programme involved white singers blacking their faces to sing songs (such as spirituals) that had been associated with slavery. The shift in cultural sensitivity means that this practice is now considered abhorrent and at odds with cultural values that respect people and their ethnicity. Actors playing the role of communicatively vulnerable people may be viewed in a similar light in future generations. Actors lack the genuine cultural knowledge of communication styles and power differentials that people from vulnerable cultural groups have. Whilst there are many organisations that could work effectively to support vulnerable service users to have a meaningful role in health and social care training, it is the professional organisation that holds the power, the budget and determines where and how it spends its money on education. Bringing in articulate service users who do not need a great deal of support may be a cheaper option (and means of ticking the service user involvement box) than paying external organisations to support willing (but potentially vulnerable) service users to access educational settings. The role of the service user now extends to involvement in training, but the role expectations may still be shaped by professionals who come from the dominant, word-based culture. Use Box 7.4 to consider whether your training has included training by people who find words hard, and the potential reasons for this. The traditional cultural view of health and social care professionals and service user roles is outlined in Figure 7.1:

Student 3:	I think the role play has limitations and it would reach limitations with this topic.
Student 1:	I think the role play especially because people … are not sure how to act if they're (playing) a patient … and it's not the same as having a real person sat in front of you.

Communicate2U quotation 7.3: The limitations of role play

Professional	Service User
A specialist who maintains a professional distance but shows a degree of emotional involvement to assure the service user of their interest. An expert with a range of knowledge that they will use to help the service user.	An individual who shows respect and due deference for the knowledge of the professional. A person who is expected to comply with information given, or provide the information that is requested.

Figure 7.1: Traditional health and social care roles (adapted from Goffman, 1959)

In some cultures that view is changing to one in which professionals and vulnerable service users work collaboratively; sharing each other's knowledge and expertise to achieve service user centred outcomes. However, cultural change can be difficult to achieve, and there will be many people who may either be cynical about this value from the start, or who work in organisations that do not enact collaborative working, and who therefore become cynical. You cannot always change the organisation, but you can change the way that you personally engage with service users. However, you will only do this if you feel it is important enough to invest time and effort to make your practice culturally competent with people who communicate in ways that are different to your own. The next sections will help you with this.

The Personal Setting: Appearance and Manner

Whenever you meet with someone you will be presenting a front. In your work culture, the front that you present will have been influenced by how other more experienced professionals have played the role that you now occupy, as well as by your own personal interpretation of that role. The front is made up of a number of factors that can be summarised as appearance and manner.

Appearance

Appearance includes aspects of grooming such as hair, make-up (if worn), body adornment (jewellery/tattoos/piercings), clothing and insignia (such as badges or wording on clothing). Have a go at the exercise in Box 7.5 to help you think about how you change your appearance to meet the norms associated with the roles that you occupy in different cultural settings.

Our appearance is an important part of our act, and one of the reasons that it is so crucial is because it tells others about our status in relation to them. In other words, it says something about power (Goffman, 1959). Putting on a uniform immediately lets others know that we are claiming to have some knowledge about a role, whether it be that of a nurse, cleaner or receptionist. Some uniforms will have a hierarchy: different coloured nurses' uniforms for example may denote different levels of power. Donning a uniform in a hospital setting also marks the wearer to be a member of staff, not a service user or visitor. This can help to define role boundaries and what behaviours are permitted within the setting. The association with uniform and professional role can sometimes make it more complex for professionals who don't wear uniforms but who work in uniformed settings (for example, social workers attending hospital meetings) as their role in the hierarchy appears more ambiguous (Pearson *et al.*, 2001; Timmons *et al.*, 2011). The seemingly simple act of donning clothing for work can therefore actually hide a multi-layered social history of role identity. Some professional roles consciously set out to minimise the power distance between service user and professional and may therefore select clothing that is closer to that of the service users that they interact with. Professionals may also use clothing to shape the role that they wish the service user to play, for example: night clothes for the sick role and day clothes for rehabilitation (Pratt *et al.*, 1997). Similarly, the way that hair is worn and the body is adorned may also

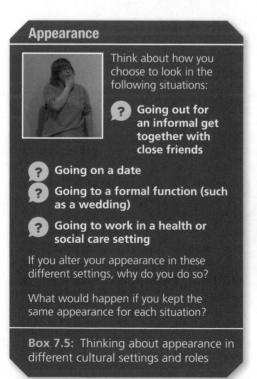

Appearance

Think about how you choose to look in the following situations:

(?) **Going out for an informal get together with close friends**

(?) **Going on a date**

(?) **Going to a formal function (such as a wedding)**

(?) **Going to work in a health or social care setting**

If you alter your appearance in these different settings, why do you do so?

What would happen if you kept the same appearance for each situation?

Box 7.5: Thinking about appearance in different cultural settings and roles help to define a role. Some jobs may require people to remove jewellery and tie hair back, or remove ties for infection control reasons (Ward 2007), but the rationale for such moves may also be perceived to have a political motivation. Such obvious outward signs of consideration towards controlling infection may be argued to be a slick way of presenting an efficient front to a gullible public who are unaware of the most efficient (but possibly less obviously visible) ways to prevent the spread of disease (Dancer, 2010). Appearances only say something about the way people wish to be perceived, not necessarily the real values that people hold beneath the surface. This point can be important to remember when you make your judgements about the service users and carers that you meet.

Service users and carers will be presenting with their own front and appearance that you will be responding to. You may see someone dressed in filthy clothing or an expensive outfit and make an automatic assumption about the type of person that they are. This does not make you a bad person – it is a natural way of trying to make sense of the huge amount of visual information that you will receive. You will initially have to fit that image into a pre-existing category that you have in your mind for someone of that appearance, even if you later receive information that requires you to modify your initial judgement (Goffman, 1959). Unlike a member of health and social care staff whose appearance has been fitted to their role during working hours, service users may occupy that title whilst wearing clothing that was actually intended for a different role. For example, a filthy, smelly person who you initially assume is a person from an impoverished background with limited access to hygiene may be a company director who has been called away from the garden at short notice to support a relative. Some care is needed not to jump to instant conclusions, but equally, the powerful information that appearance can communicate to you should not be overlooked. This is particularly the case when you work with service users who cannot use words to speak to you, and who are cared for by others. Their appearance can tell you a lot about the types of activities that they may do, or the quality of care that they receive. The information on appearance can be the starting point to explore more deeply. For example, a person who is totally dependent on others for washing and dressing who is in stained clothing that smells strongly is not in a position to make an informed choice about personal hygiene. Such an appearance may indicate that carers are not coping well, that there is a lack of care, or that the person has just recently had an accident: it is part of your job to notice potential warning signs and to follow these up. Similarly, a person who appears to be hiding bruises may in fact be telling a story that a health or social care worker needs to listen to. Patterns of bruising that could indicate too firm a grasp or strangulation may be signs of abuse, particularly when stories about how they have occurred are inconsistent (Clarke *et al.*, 1999; Fărcaş *et al.*, 2004). The current drive in countries such as the UK towards a less risk aversive view towards vulnerable service users (Dunn *et al.*, 2008) can also mean that people who previously didn't get bruised because they did little activity are now more active and at risk of minor bruising. However, suspected cases of abuse should always be followed up and dealt with in accordance with policies and procedures: an inefficient handling of suspicions can prejudice later investigations. Appearances, and how they are noted by health and social care staff, are therefore potentially very

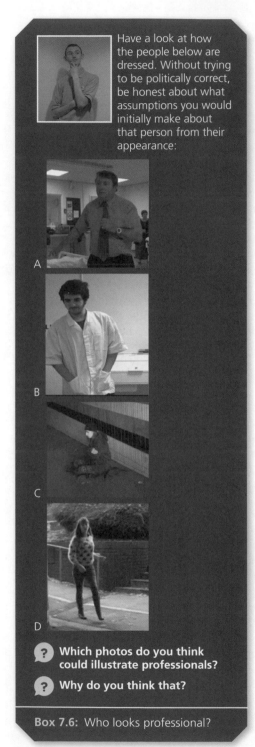

Have a look at how the people below are dressed. Without trying to be politically correct, be honest about what assumptions you would initially make about that person from their appearance:

A

B

C

D

? Which photos do you think could illustrate professionals?

? Why do you think that?

Box 7.6: Who looks professional?

powerful communication tools. The way in which service users and carers note the appearance of health and social care staff can also be a powerful factor in communication.

You may have no choice over the clothing that you wear in your work role, and limited control as to how you are permitted to wear your hair or use body adornment. You may be in a position to consciously select how you look, in which case you may consciously opt to include little touches that emphasise your professional distance or minimise it. Whichever the case, it is important to recognise that your appearance will be sending a message to service users. Some may consciously be aware of the power that your appearance, uniform or badge conveys, and note how efficient or approachable you look. Others may unconsciously respond to your look. The reactions of service users and carers may be based on experiences with other professionals who looked similar to you. If their experiences have been positive, you may be lucky: they will be starting the interaction with a positive view of you and the profession that you embody. If they have previously had poor experiences, you may have to do a lot of work to initially overcome their unease. One of the major ways in which you can achieve this is by your manner.

Manner

Manner (Goffman, 1959) links with the concept of key or tone (Hymes, 2005), which was a component of communication explored in Chapter 3. It is the way that we act to portray ourselves to others in a way that matches our perceived values. When we meet with others we may wish to come across as serious, caring, professional, informal or any other one of a host of adjectives that describe the performance that we are about to engage in. Manner is linked to both the characteristics of the individual and the setting in which the performance occurs. For example, you may have a natural tendency towards formality or informality, but you will have to modify this according to the cultural environment in which your interactions take place. Some of you looking at picture B in Box 7.6 above may have noted the hands in the pockets stance of the healthcare professional and thought it looked too informal or unprofessional for someone in that role. Manner is shown through a range of different communication components: body language, tone of voice, facial expression and the types of words and phrases that are used – aspects of communication that were covered in Chapters 3 to 5. Have a go at the exercise in Box 7.7 to identify words that you feel are associated with the manner that people in your profession should be portraying when engaging with service users. Then have a go at identifying words that you feel service users should be portraying when they engage with professionals.

> ### Manner
>
>
> Go online and watch the drama produced by Communicate2U that illustrates how your manner affects how you are viewed by service users. The short, humorous piece makes a serious point: manner is important!
>
> **Box 7.7:** Mind your manners

One of the skills that is required when performing is that of supressing immediate emotions that may conflict with audience expectations of the role (Goffman, 1959). Your role as a caring professional means it would be inappropriate to show feelings such as anger or disgust towards a service user or carer. However, there may well be occasions when this is your natural first response. Your natural emotion has to be transformed into an intellectualised empathic response that requires a cognitive effort (Davis, 1983). Service users and carers too will often have an image of their role and this will be shaped by cultural influences. For example, even something as seemingly basic as how we experience pain and how acceptable it is to show that to others can vary widely at the national level of culture (Callister, 2003). At other cultural levels, this same concept applies: if you dropped something heavy on your foot during an interview for an important job you would probably respond in quite a different way to if you were at home. Most of us have experienced the role of service user in health care settings, and we have acts that will be based on our own cultural experiences. When you go to the doctor as a patient you will have an image of how you are expected to behave, and may be conscious of a choice of performances to select from. You could be the apologetic patient, sorry to take up the doctor's time; the professional patient who wishes to have a collaborative discussion about how treatment should progress, or the really ill patient who requires urgent responses to their problems and wants the doctor to take on the responsibility for care. You may find that you use different acts in different situations or settings.

People who are under stress, or who lack the cognitive ability to supress the initial emotional response will not necessarily play the role that others may expect of them. A service user who shows raw, unmodified emotion or who doesn't listen and act on professional advice may not match the act that professionals have come to expect from those that they work with. Professionals may not know how to respond in such situations, and when there is a conflict of cultural styles the natural response is to do even more of the same (Tannen, 2005). This could result in the professional becoming more distant, which in turn may make the service user more emotional. This can lead to both parties in an interaction feeling uncomfortable. Toni, below, illustrates this as she describes how health and social care professionals who come into a special school often react when they meet children whose communication is through forms of behaviour that may seem unusual to a newcomer:

(The professionals are) Often alarmed. Often very out of their depth, that they have a specialism ... They know what they can do, but they're faced with a young person who isn't reacting how the majority of young people act. And so, they don't have the skills to deal with that, and then all their humanistic skills kind of almost desert them, is what I'd say. (Toni)

Communicate2U quotation 7.4: Toni sees professionals' discomfort when visiting a special school

The professional who is faced with a service user who does not use words can revert to purely talking to staff to get their message across, thereby ignoring the person who is the subject of their intervention. Not only do they upset both service user and carer, they also come across as lacking in humanity. If professionals wish to come across as caring to the most vulnerable of communicators, their act has to include a performance that works with people who communicate predominantly on an emotional level. The problem here is that humans are predisposed to misinterpreting emotions at the best of times. If you are looking thoughtful, preoccupied or tired this could be misinterpreted as being annoyed or angry. It is only the basic emotions such as happiness, anger, sadness and disgust that are universally recognised across cultures. Therefore, to reduce the chances of your manner being interpreted as uninterested or hostile, you will need to work on approaching the majority of interactions with a friendly smile – even if the act may feel insincere. This, however, has to be followed up by a very sincere attempt to communicate in a way that is accessible to the service user. People who can't use words are highly sensitive to emotional communication from you and will pick up straight away if you are too worried to, or can't be bothered to, make a genuine effort to communicate with them.

Professional Scripts

Professional scripts are ritualised ways of interacting that you will learn as you become familiar with your role. If they are to be inclusive you will need to understand what your script is and, in addition, you will need to have the following skills:

- Flexibility
- Openness
- Tolerance for differences
- Ability to cope with ambiguity
- Creativity in seeking new ways to communicate
- Willingness to get involved
- Sensitivity to the underlying emotional message

(Chen *et al.*, 1996a; Devito, 1997; Jandt, 2007)

If you have undertaken the practical exercises within this book and looked at the films created by the cultural experts in alternative communication forms you should by now recognise these skills in yourself. You will be ready to transfer the skills to your professional role. If you haven't and have focused on the written, academic word, you will have missed the main point of this text, and are advised to go back and have a real go at challenging your cultural conditioning. The final sections will support you to explore ways of examining your professional scripts and making them more inclusive for people who do not communicate well with the words that you are used to using in your professional role. It will go through some of the stages that are common to the encounters that service users experience when engaging with professional staff.

THE INVITATION TO MEET

Generic Health and Social Care Trust

Dear Service User,

I am writing to invite you to attend an appointment to discuss your issues with our hospital and community support team. You will need to come to:

The Town Centre, Central Lane, ZZZ123

On Thursday 15th July at 2pm

A map is shown on the reverse side of this letter.

Please ensure that you bring with you copies of any recent letters that you have received from our team. If you have any additional needs, please let us know in advance using the contact details at the bottom of this letter.

Here at Generic Health and Social Care Trust we are committed to providing you with the highest quality and most compassionate care. At Generic Health and Social Care Trust, we aim to create an atmosphere of partnership working that is underpinned by our recognition of your right to client centred treatment.

The Generic Health and Social Care Trust values of caring, respect, integrity, collaboration and excellence are ones that we constantly strive to improve. We welcome feedback on our services and look forward to meeting with you to explore how we can better meet our service aims.

Best wishes,

A Professional

Figure 7.2: An example of a standard letter sent to service users

If you are currently working in a health and social care setting, have a look at a standard letter that is sent out to your service users. If you don't have access to a letter, look at the example above, or think back to a time when you have been sent a letter for an appointment. Now think about how accessible the letter shown above would be for the following populations:

- People who don't have English as a first language
- People who have a reading ability below that required to read a story to a child aged around 9 years
- People with a learning disability
- People with dementia who are finding it difficult to concentrate
- People with visual impairment
- Any person who finds words hard, for whatever reason

People are often ashamed if they cannot read information that is sent to them. They may not ask for help and may be unaware of the content of your communication. It is your job as a culturally aware professional to ensure that your communication is effective. If people fail to attend appointments, there can be a tendency for health and social care staff to assume that it is because they do not wish to come and that they are unappreciative of the help that is being offered. They blame the other for the communication error (Jandt, 2007). From an intercultural communication perspective, a better stance would be to wonder what it was about the communication that deterred or prevented them from attending. The quotation from Malcolm, who has supported many young people and families through social care meetings, illustrates this point:

... so that any letters that come, for instance, which are often just total gobbledegook to families, particularly families that are illiterate in the first place and can't read. And I've known many instances of people not turning up to meetings, and you say, well, why aren't they here? Well, we've sent a letter. But the family can't read ... they (the professional) *didn't even know that simple fact.* (Malcolm, Communicate2U)

Communicate2U quotation 7.5: Malcolm explains the impact of poor professional communication on attendance at meetings

Letters are often the first point of contact between a service user and a service. They can set the tone for an encounter before professionals and service users meet. A service user who has had a letter that is hard to understand may be fearful as to how they will cope with a meeting with the person who sent it, or worse still, they may not understand that they are being offered an appointment. Professional staff are culturally conditioned to using words and may feel uncomfortable at changing the communicative style to a simpler register for fear that it is treating end users like a child (Ochs, 1993). However, a failure to offer an alternative, more accessible version of a letter alongside the written version can result in non-attendance (Gordon *et al.*, 2002). Initiatives such as accessible information packs and follow up phone calls to confirm appointments (Hardy *et al.*, 2001) or short text messages to remind people to attend (Liew *et al.*, 2009) can have a big impact on the accessibility and effectiveness of services. Compare the letter above with the one in Figure 7.3:

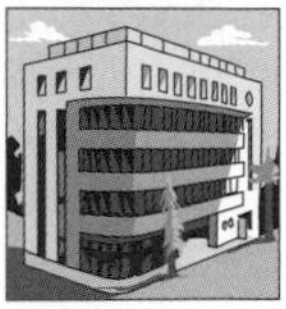	My name is Annette I work with the generic Trust I work at the Town Centre
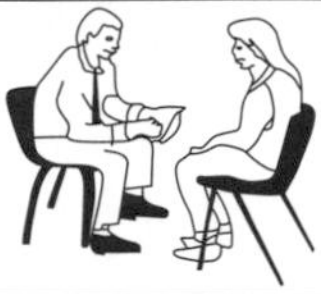	Your doctor has asked you to come to talk with me I'd like to help make things better
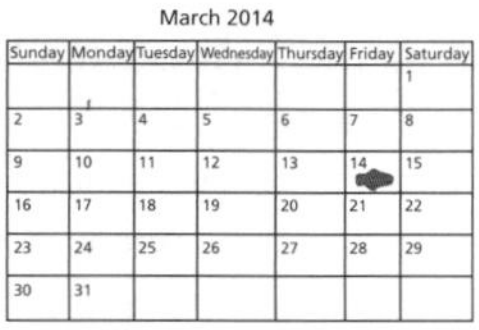	I'd like to meet you on Friday 14th March
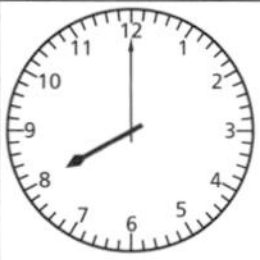	At 8 o'clock in the morning
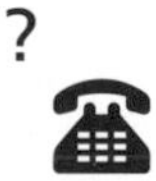 ? 	If you have any questions, ring me on this number: 0000 555 4567
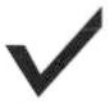 ✔ Yes I can come 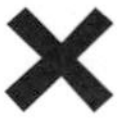 ✘ No I can't come	I will phone you to see if you can come If you want to make it a different time or day, that is ok

Figure 7.3: An example of an attempt at an easy read letter

Principles for making written material more accessible for everyone include:

- Use clear pictures at the left hand side of the page. This shows that they are important
- Use pictures of the real buildings (and if possible the real people) if inviting service users to specific places
- Make sure that pictures link clearly to the words that you use
- Write in short sentences – one idea per sentence
- One line per sentence
- Use simple words (but be aware that some words have more than one meaning – pictures help here too)
- Use numbers (e.g. 8) rather than words (eight)
- Use an easy to read font such as Ariel, in 16 point (Mencap, nd)

This approach combined with a follow up phone call to back up all letters sent out may sound a cumbersome procedure, but may actually save time that is wasted on missed appointments. If both formats of letters are sent out it also sends a very powerful message to service users and carers: we are flexible in our communication, we want to communicate well with you and we are putting our values into action. A wordy letter that talks about quality and partnership working, yet excludes vulnerable people is not achieving this effect. Multi-modal communication – using more than one form at the same time – increases the chances of communication being effective (Goldbart et al., 2010). These principles apply whether the format is on paper, in the environment or in face to face encounters as shown below.

THE INITIAL MEETING

Assuming that people have read the letter, had the phone call and decided that you are approachable enough to follow up on the invitation, the next step will be them attending for an appointment. They will have to find you. The principles of clear communication outlined above need to extend to information that is sent to help people find your place of work. Maps can be difficult to follow: pictures of the location, the nearest train station and bus stops can help to improve the chances of someone making it to the appointment. An example of a visual map is shown in Figure 7.4.

Getting to City Hospital from the train station

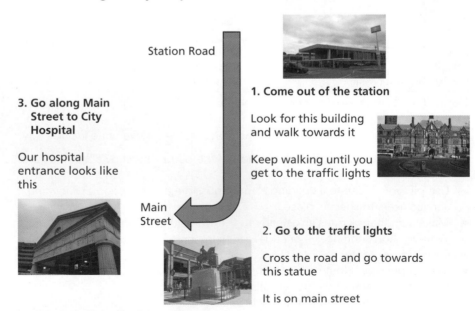

Station Road

3. Go along Main Street to City Hospital

Our hospital entrance looks like this

Main Street

1. Come out of the station

Look for this building and walk towards it

Keep walking until you get to the traffic lights

2. Go to the traffic lights

Cross the road and go towards this statue

It is on main street

Figure 7.4: Example of a visual map

Colour coding, use of icons and contrasts between signs and backgrounds can all improve location finding:

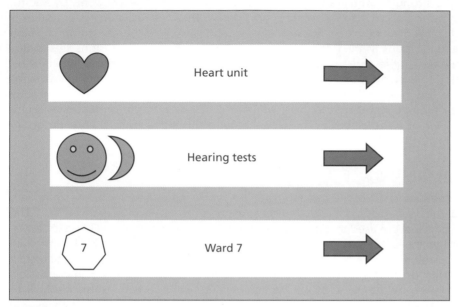

Figure 7.5: Simplified sign with symbols

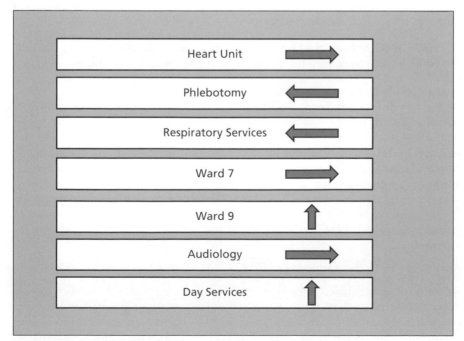

Figure 7.6: Sign without symbols

Have a look at the two signboards shown in Figures 7.5 and 7.6 and consider which system you would prefer to have in place if you had to direct people who struggled with reading English. Signs can be simplified not only by adding in symbols, but also by splitting up signs so that not too much information is displayed in one place. For example, locations to the right may go on one sign and locations to the left on a separate sign. If the letters and signage systems are accessible and a phone call has been made to follow up the initial invitation to account for poor postal systems, the service user may make it as far as the first meeting. The opening few moments of an interaction can set the tone for the encounter that follows, whether it occurs with the professional themselves or a receptionist. Therefore, getting this stage right is very important (Devito, 1997).

The Greeting

Greetings can be viewed as a ritual; a highly patterned exchange that both parties generally understand and can respond to in kind (Goffman, 1981). The words that are used to identify ourselves in relation to others are linked to power. When meeting a service user or carer for the first time, you will have to introduce yourself if you are to be viewed as polite. You may choose to use a title such as Mr/Mrs/Ms/Dr and surname, or may choose to say your first name (possibly followed by the name of our profession). You will also have to decide how to address the person you are meeting (Danziger, 1976). As the professional, you will tend to initiate the greeting and will have the greater power to set the tone for how distant or close the power distance between yourself and the other person is, as shown in the examples below:

A)   Hello, Fred, my name is Dr Roebuck and I'm your therapist
B)   Hello, my name is Annette, I'm your therapist. What's your name?

In example A, the therapist assumes a dominant stance by using a first name for the service user, and emphasises her power in the relationship by using the honorific 'Dr' for her own name. In example B, the power distance is minimised by the use of the less formal first name, and by handing the power to the service user to determine how they would prefer to label themselves. The ritualistic nature of greetings also explains why people can feel justifiably angry if service users are not given a direct personal greeting: their existence as a human being who is worthy of a basic acknowledgment is denied. Whilst greetings can actually be quite complex, and different situations may require different degrees of formality (Danziger, 1976; Goffman, 1981), there is one basic rule that should be followed:

Always speak to the service user first

As the quotation below illustrates, even if the service user has no speech, greeting someone shows that you are viewing them as a communicating human being. Walter has very limited speech and his parents interpret his non-verbal communication and often speak on his behalf. Both Walter and his parents appreciate staff speaking to him first, as his mother Trudy explains:

> *Well, obviously, we tend to be his spokesperson. But we regularly go to the diabetic clinic who all know him pretty well now and they're fantastic because I have never been made to feel ... you know, they've always greeted him first, you know. (they say) "hello, Walter" (Trudy)*

Communicate2U quotation 7.6: Trudy explains the importance of staff greeting her non-verbal son by name

There may be occasions when you greet the service user, and carers take that opportunity to inform you that the person cannot talk back to you. Thank them for that information, but be sure then to adapt your communication to be inclusive during all the stages of the interaction that follows.

Each profession and each cultural setting will have patterns that are followed when service users engage with services. This may be obvious (such as a formal hospital admission process) or hidden (such as the ways in which service users are asked to make choices in a social care settings (Antaki *et al.*, 2008; Antaki *et al.*, 2009; Antaki *et al.*, 2007c)). When you first enter a profession or new job, many of these patterns will seem unfamiliar and you will need to consciously learn them. Remembering these experiences can be vitally important, because at that stage you are a newcomer to the culture. That helps you to see what it may be like for a cultural outsider. Over time you will become culturally blind to many aspects of the interactions that other people will find strange and unfamiliar. You may well be very comfortable in asking strangers to give you very personal information, or undress for you. For the person on the receiving end, that can be very new and upsetting. You will use verbal short cuts and expect others to know your meaning (Goffman, 1981). For example, you may ask someone how they are. In reality you want them to tell you what problems they have that need your attention; you may become impatient if they then go on to give you what you deem to be irrelevant information about how upset they are with because the kids were fighting in the car on the way to the appointment. You will not be communicating as clearly as you think you are to others because you will have adapted to the new cultural norm of your profession and organisation. Have a go at the exercise in Box 7.8 to explore the kinds of interaction rituals that are associated with your profession. If you have trouble seeing them, try them out on someone who doesn't know your profession and get feedback from them on how it feels; in other words start to value the views of people from outside of your own culture in order to become more culturally competent.

A New Ritual for Interactions: Cultural Sensitivity and Multi-Modal Communication

If you have read the chapters on words (Chapter 3), the musical aspects of speech (Chapter 4) and non-verbal communication (Chapter 5) you should by now understand that you are already a culturally versatile communicator who has a wide repertoire of communication styles at your fingertips. If you haven't, you need to at least go back and do some of the practical exercises. You now need to understand that the skills that you have in other cultural settings such as the family and social groups are important in your professional role too. With family and friends you tend to get quite good at attending to the emotional messages that they send; if you don't, relationships often break down. In your professional role, there is often a lot of factual information to gain and convey, but if the emotional message is ignored, communication breakdown can occur in this setting too (Kruijver *et al.*, 2001). In Chapter 2, you were introduced to the idea that as a professional, you hold the balance of power in communication exchanges with service users and carers. As the book has progressed, you will have hopefully gained a much clearer idea as to what forms that power takes in all aspects of communication: the way that you use your body language, voice and environment. In comparison to the majority of service users and carers, whatever their background, you are privileged and powerful when in your professional role.

Your Professional Rituals

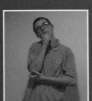

Think about your usual professional script when you meet service users. This may include ritualised stages such as:

- Initial interviews
- Counselling
- Assessment
- Carrying out examinations

- Explaining how systems (such as benefit payments) work
- Asking people to make choices about their lives and daily routines (Antaki *et al.*, 2008; Antaki *et al.*, 2007a; Finlay *et al.*, 2008a; Finlay *et al.*, 2008b; Finlay *et al.*, 2008c)
- Discharge from services

? **What kind of adaptations would you need to make to these stages to make them more accessible to people who find words hard?**

? **Would you need to adapt paperwork to include easy read versions of information?**

? **Would you need props or objects to show people your ideas?**

? **Would you need pictures?**

? **Could you act out things to show people what you mean?**

? **Could you be creative and develop videos to show people instead of telling them?**

? **If you don't do these things, who will?**

? **What would be the impact on vulnerable service users if these adaptations were not done?**

Box 7.8: Adapting your professional rituals

If you retain power by clinging to ways of communicating that suit your own personal or professional style, you run the risk of inadvertently harming vulnerable service users. If, however, you adapt your communication style so that it mirrors the preferred style of the service user, then you are more likely to meet professional aims of caring, compassion and client-centred care (to name but a few). You are reminded that the way to do this is to notice and address power imbalances and communication styles. If words are hard for your communication partner, make sure you use good body language, tone of voice, pictures or objects to back up what you are saying. If a person doesn't use words at all but uses sounds or actions – learn what these mean from someone who knows them well and mirror them. If you are talking over someone, give them more time and mirror their speed of talking.

All of us may be in a position at some point in our lives when we need support from health or social care staff. Those times will often be ones that are stressful to us, and we may struggle to concentrate and communicate as well as we do at other times. We may need staff to slow down to let us take things in. We may need information to be backed up in a user friendly, written format to help us remember what has been said. We are all potentially communicatively vulnerable service users to some degree. Therefore improving your intercultural communication will not only benefit people with a learning disability, dementia, mental health needs or sensory needs to name but a few marginalised client groups. *Get it right for the most vulnerable communicators, and you get it right for everyone.*

The key to achieving this is summarised in Figure 7.7.

1. Remember that EVERYONE COMMUNICATES and it is your job to ADAPT your communication style to suit

2. LOOK for communication and MIRROR the communication style of the other person

3. Try to understand the EMOTION behind the behaviour

4. Use a MIXTURE of STRATEGIES (body language/pictures/objects) as a routine strategy to back up your words

5. CHECK BACK UNDERSTANDING – explain that you may not always communicate well and the only way you can tell if you have done a good job is by asking the person to TELL or SHOW you what you have said

6. SEEK support from experts when needed, but always have a go at basic communication yourself

Figure 7.7: Basic rules for good intercultural communication in health and social care

This will not come naturally to everyone. You may need to work at the strategies. You may also need to ensure that the places in which you work have the props that you need to perform this type of interaction: pictures of routinely referred to objects, people or services for example. You may still need to communicate complex factual information to carers or support workers, but this should be followed up by a short, accessible summary of key points at frequent intervals.

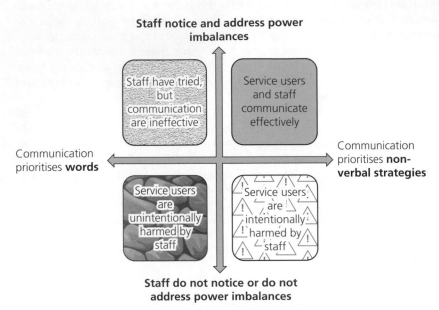

Figure 7.8: Mapping the impact of staff communication strategies on vulnerable service users

The model that was introduced in Chapter 2 and is shown again here in Figure 7.8 can be used to help you quickly map whether you are working in a way that is likely to do harm or good to vulnerable people. Using the strategies summarised in Figure 7.7 puts you in the smooth zone as you notice the inherent power imbalance between yourself and people who find words hard and use non-word-based strategies instead. If you don't make these adaptations then you run the risk of being an ineffective communicator with vulnerable people and not listening to their needs (bumpy zone) unintentionally harming people (rocky zone). It is hoped that someone who has been motivated enough to read this far will not be a person who deliberately uses the power to physically harm vulnerable people (danger zone). Your own heightened cultural sensitivity to more effective communication with vulnerable people may also help you to note cases in which carers or support workers do not use such strategies themselves when communicating with vulnerable people. These are the individuals who are at the greatest risk of all. If vulnerable people have no one who can see their emotional communication and respond appropriately to their needs, they will remain isolated in a world that is dominated by words.

CHAPTER SUMMARY

There are many different approaches to viewing communication with vulnerable people, but this book has argued that thinking of it in intercultural terms has a number of factors that make it worth trying. It's nothing new – we already have the skills and we often use them in other aspects of our lives. Therefore, with a little bit of thought and practice, it shouldn't be hard to transfer these basic methods to communicating with people who we may feel are difficult or impossible to communicate with. This approach also means that there is no excuse for failing to communicate with all service users – both the articulate ones and those who don't use words well. If communication seems difficult or seems to be going wrong, ask yourself the following questions:

- What are the cultural values and communication styles of the other person?
- How do they differ from my own?
- Am I dominating the interaction by using the form of communication that I'm most comfortable with?
- What can I do to adapt my form of communication so that it matches their style more closely?
- If I don't adapt – how could this affect the service user?

A new script for health and social care staff

On the companion website, the key themes of this book are summarised in two different formats.

You Talk to Your Dog is a song that highlights how talking to non-verbal animals or objects is a cultural norm, yet communicating with non-verbal service users is a skill that many staff lack. Watch the video to learn how this affects vulnerable people, and learn the simple things you can do to alter your script to one that is inclusive.

The *Sea of Words* ballet uses no spoken words at all to communicate the same themes to you. It uses dance as a communicative medium since this is a format that the members of Freefall Dance Company are experts in. As you watch the ballet think back to your assumptions about Jeff in Chapter 1 and see if your thinking has developed during the course of reading this book.

Box 7.9: A new script for health and social care summarised in musical and dance-based formats

These are not complex questions, but in asking them you are making an important shift. Instead of blaming the other person for their communicative incompetence, you are turning into a cultural detective who is actively looking for clues to improve their own communication performance. Your professional script can then develop to include simple techniques that you would naturally use with someone from another culture: using pictures, gestures and facial expressions instead of words. As a baseline, you should ensure that you always aim to communicate at an emotional level with every service user and carer you come into contact with in your job. You will not always get things right. You will make mistakes; you'll try a technique one time and it will work, only to find that the next time it doesn't. Coping with ambiguity and errors is nothing new – it is what communication is all about (Berger *et al.*, 1969; Devito, 1997). To cope with this you can use trial and error – tentatively try out a way of communicating. Look to see how the other person is responding and adapt your style if it doesn't seem to be working. You will at least be seeing the communicatively vulnerable person as an individual who is worthy of your time and attention, and who has needs that you are seeking to address. You will be trying to give them the same kind of attention that you would give to any other person in need of your help. In doing so, you reduce the risk of vulnerable service users being harmed because their basic needs have been overlooked. In the past such abuses were routine but overlooked. In many health and social care cultures, however, they are no longer tolerated, and staff have to adapt their performance or run the risk of spending valuable time in managing complaints and investigations. There has been a cultural shift in how vulnerable people are viewed in health and social care environments, and an expectation that they should receive equitable treatment. It is hoped that this book has given you an additional tool in your communication toolbox to help you to shape the culture to one that is inclusive of all people who require support from health and social care staff.

EASY READ CHAPTER SUMMARY

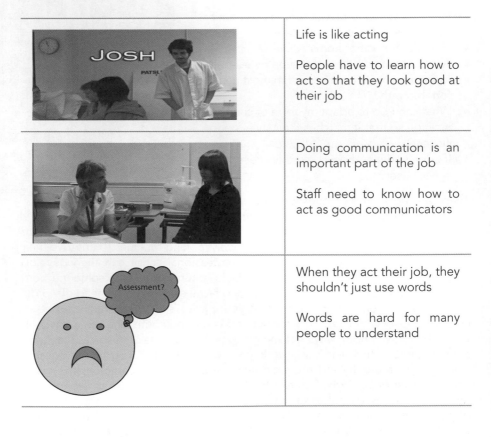

	Life is like acting
	People have to learn how to act so that they look good at their job
	Doing communication is an important part of the job
	Staff need to know how to act as good communicators
	When they act their job, they shouldn't just use words
	Words are hard for many people to understand

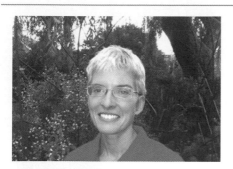

They shouldn't just talk

They also need to:

Look friendly

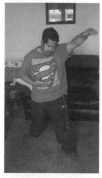

Use actions to show us what they mean

Use pictures to help us understand what they say

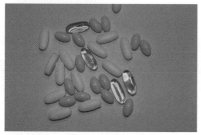

Tablet

Or

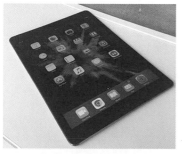

Tablet

Show us how things work instead of just telling us

	My name is Annette I work with the generic Trust I work at the Town Centre
	Your doctor has asked you to come to talk with me I'd like to help make things better
March 2014	I'd like to meet you on Friday 14th March
	At 8 o'clock in the morning
?	If you have any questions, ring me on this number: 0000 555 4567
✓ Yes I can come ✗ No I can't come	I will phone you to see if you can come If you want to make it a different time or day, that is ok

They need to write letters that are easy to understand

Letters should have pictures as well as words

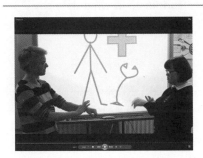

People who find words hard also have good ways of communicating

The ways of communicating may be different

so

Staff need to learn from us

GLOSSARY OF TERMS

Adaptors
: Adaptors are movements that we engage in when we respond to an inner drive (such as an itch).

Affect displays
: Affect displays are those body movements that directly convey the emotional message.

Agency
: Agency is a type of power. It links to the motivations that drive individuals to act in the way that they do, and the degree of freedom that they have to act upon those drives.

Appearance
: Appearance includes aspects of grooming such as hair, make-up (if worn), body adornment (jewellery/tattoos/piercings), clothing and insignia (such as badges or wording on clothing).

Argot
: Argot is a term to describe the specialised language systems that are used by members of a group. Knowing and using the words appropriately demonstrates group membership.

Bias
: Bias is a mechanism that more powerful people can use to limit the choices available to the less powerful. An example of bias is leaving items off an agenda so they do not get discussed.

Collectivist culture
: In a collectivist culture the emphasis is on relationships between people, and individual needs may be subsumed into a goal that benefits wider society.

Communication
: Effective communication with vulnerable people occurs when the most powerful communicator within an exchange acknowledges and responds to the emotional (and if present, factual) message sent in a manner that is consistent with the cultural style of the least powerful communicator.

Cultural norms
: Cultural norms are the patterns of behaviour and values that people who have regular contact with each other develop. They are based upon dimensions of culture.

Cultural values
: Cultural values are beliefs that are held by pivotal members of that culture and by a majority of its members.

Culture
: Culture is the normative patterns of behaviour and communication that are developed over time and enacted by people who share, or are affected by, common values and beliefs.

Culture clash	A culture clash can occur when people from different cultural backgrounds meet. If they fail to recognise that they have different norms for interaction, each assumes that the other person is a poor communicator. Negative emotions result.
Culture shock	Culture shock can occur when a person spends time living in a culture that is very different to their own. They experience disorientation and distress because of the hidden cultural differences.
Dimensions of culture	Dimensions of culture are the underlying patterns that influence how people from a cultural group behave and communicate. Dimensions include considerations of context, individualism and collectivism, power, uncertainty avoidance, time orientation and masculinity/femininity.
Dominant culture	The cultural group that has the power to set the norms within an interaction is the dominant culture. For example, health and social care staff are members of the dominant culture when they interact with service users.
Emblems	Emblems are movements that can be directly translated into words (Devito, 1997).
Exclusive communication	Exclusive communication occurs when the meaning communicated is not accessible to all members of an interaction. This may happen intentionally, or unintentionally.
Formal learning	Formal learning is gained from an authority figure who uses example or punishment to teach. Formal knowledge is linked to strong emotions and is resistant to change.
Generative view of power	If you have a generative view of power you believe that sharing power with others generates more power overall.
Haptics	A technical term used to describe the use of touch within communication.
High context culture	A high context culture is one in which the relationship between the communication partners and background knowledge (for example, about the partner's status) is more important than the word-based message. The key communication aim is to maintain harmonious relationships.
High uncertainty avoidance cultures	High uncertainty avoidance cultures tend towards security seeking acts that may have a more aggressive tone, and members can be emotional and intolerant.
Inclusive communication	Inclusive communication occurs when the meaning communicated is accessible to all members of an interaction.
Individualist culture	In an individualist culture, the individual and their immediate family are of primary importance. Other parties have minimal priority and there is competition between individuals.
Informal learning	Informal learning is unconsciously gained from observation of others and the rules associated with what is learned are hidden and pervasive.

Intercultural competence	Intercultural competence is the ability to communicate effectively across cultures of any level. A person who recognises that communication difficulties may be caused by differing cultural norms and who takes the initiative to address these differences is demonstrating intercultural competence.
Kinesics	A technical term used to describe the role of movement and gesture within interpersonal communication.
Low context culture	A low context culture is one in which the message that is conveyed through words is more important than background knowledge about communication partners. The key communication aim is to convey a clear and unambiguous message.
Low uncertainty avoidance	People in low uncertainty avoidance cultures tend to be more relaxed and comfortable with taking risks.
Manner	Manner is the way that we act to portray ourselves to others in a way that matches our perceived values. Manner is linked to both the characteristics of the individual and the setting in which the performance occurs.
Mirroring	Mirroring occurs when one communication partner matches the body language and musical aspects of speech of the other.
Non-dominant culture	The cultural group that has less power to set the norms within an interaction is the non-dominant culture. For example, service users with additional communication needs may have ways of communicating that can be viewed as different to the word-based culture of health and social care, and they are therefore non-dominant.
Paralanguage	Paralanguage is a term used to describe the musical components of speech such as pitch, tone, pace and timing.
Polysemy	Words that have many different meanings.
Professional performance scripts	Ritualised ways of interacting with others that professionals learn as they become familiar with their roles.
Prosody	Prosody is a term used to describe the musical components of speech such as pitch, tone and timing.
Proxemics	A term used to describe the way that the distance between people impacts upon an interpersonal exchange.
Regulators	Regulators are the movements (and sounds) that we use to try to control the person who is interacting with us (Devito, 1997).
Role sincerity	The degree to which an individual believes in the values associated with the role that they are playing.
Structure	Structure is a term used to describe the forces within organisations or cultures that constrain an individual's use of power.
Technical learning	Technical learning occurs when expert members of a culture explicitly pass on their knowledge to novices in a structured manner (for example, during a lecture or within a

	book). Technical learning tends to have a limited emotional component.
Vocal qualifiers	Vocal qualifiers are the seemingly nonsensical sounds that we use (for example, uh oh). They are not words, but they communicate emotional meaning.
Zero sum view of power	If you have a zero sum view of power you believe that giving some power to others diminishes the amount of power that you hold.

REFERENCES

Adolphs R, Sears L, Piven J (2001). Abnormal processing of social information from faces in autism. *Journal Of Cognitive Neuroscience* **13**(2): 232–240.

Altman I (1975). *The Environment and Social Behavior: Privacy, Personal Space, Territory, and Crowding*. Brooks/Cole Publishing Company: California.

Andelson JG (2002). Coming together and breaking apart: Sociogenesis and schismogenesis in intentional communities. *Intentional Community: An Anthropological Perspective*: 131–152.

Andersen PA, Leibowitz K (1978). The development and nature of the construct touch avoidance. *Environmental psychology and nonverbal behavior* **3**(2): 89–106.

Antaki C, Finlay W, Walton C, Pate L (2008). Offering choices to people with intellectual disabilities: An interactional study. *Journal of Intellectual Disability Research* **52**(12): 1165–1175.

Antaki C, Finlay WML, Walton C (2009). Choices for people with intellectual disabilities: Official discourse and everyday practice. *Journal of Policy and Practice in Intellectual Disabilities* **6**(4): 260–266.

Antaki C, Finlay WML, Walton C (2007a). Conversational shaping: Staff members' solicitation of talk from people with an intellectual impairment. *Qualitative Health Research* **17**(10): 1403–1414.

Antaki C, Finlay WML, Walton C (2007b). The staff are your friends: Intellectually disabled identities in official discourse and interactional practice. *British Journal of Social Psychology* **46**(1): 1–18.

Antaki C, Walton C, Finlay WML (2007c). How proposing an activity to a person with an intellectual disability can imply a limited identity. *Discourse & Society* **18**(4): 393–410.

Apter B (2014). Foucauldian Iterative Learning Conversations – an example of organisational change: developing conjoint-work between EPs and social workers. *Educational Psychology in Practice* **30**(4): 331–346.

Aquino AT, Lee SS (2000). The use of nonerotic touch with children: Ethical and developmental considerations. *Journal of Psychotherapy in Independent Practice* **1**(3): 17–30.

Argyle M (2013). *Bodily Communication (Second Edition)*. Routledge: New York.

Argyle M, Dean J (1965). Eye-contact, distance and affiliation. *Sociometry*: 289–304.

Arif-Rahu M, Grap MJ (2010). Facial expression and pain in the critically ill non-communicative patient: State of science review. *Intensive and Critical Care Nursing* **26**(6): 343–352.

Atkinson D, Ingham N, Welshman J (2005). Change....and continuity. In: *Witnesses to Change: Families, Learning Difficulties and History.*, Rolph S, Atkinson D, Nind M, Walmsley J (eds). Kidderminster: BILD.

Atkinson D, Jackson M, Walmsley J (2000). Introduction: Methods and themes. In: *Forgotten Lives: Exploring the History of Learning Disability*, Atkinson D, Jackson M, Walmsley J (eds). BILD: Kidderminster.

Avery P (2007). *Luke's Three Dimensional Model of Power Reduc: Is It Still Compelling?* Gale, Cenage Learning: Florida.

Ayotte J, Peretz I, Hyde K (2002). Congenital amusia: A group study of adults afflicted with a music-specific disorder. *Brain: A Journal of Neurology* **125**(2): 238–251.

Ayres J (1979). *Sensory Integration and the Child*. Western Psychological Services: LA.

Baccarani C, Ugolini M (2014). A 5 Senses Perspective to Quality in Hospitals. *Toulon-Verona Conference 'Excellence in Services'*.

Bachrach P, Baratz MS (1963). Decisions and non decisions. *American Political Science Review* **57**.

Bachrach P, Baratz MS (1962). The two faces of power. *American Political Science Review* **56**.

Back AL, Bauer-Wu SM, Rushton CH, Halifax J (2009). Compassionate silence in the patient–clinician encounter: a contemplative approach. *Journal of Palliative Medicine* **12**(12): 1113–1117.

Bailey B (2005). Multiple identities among Dominican Americans. In: Kiesling SF, Bratt-Paulston C. *Intercultural Discourse and Communication*. Malden, CA; Oxford; Victoria: Blackwell Publishing.

Balandin S, Hemsley B, Sigafoos J, Green V (2007a). Communicating with nurses: The experiences of 10 adults with cerebral palsy and complex communication needs. *Applied Nursing Research* **20**(2): 56–62.

Bandura A (1971). *Social Learning Theory*. General Learning Press: New York.

Bard MR, Goettler CE, Schenarts PJ, Collins BA, Toschlog EA, Sagraves SG, *et al.* (2004). Language barrier leads to the unnecessary intubation of trauma patients. *The American Surgeon* **70**(9): 783–786.

Barna LM (1997). Stumbling blocks in intercultual communication. In: *Intercultural Communication: A Reader*, Samovar LA, Porter RE (eds). Belmont, CA: Wadsworth.

Barnes M, Bowl K (2001). *Taking Over the Asylum – Empowerment and Mental Health*. Palgrave: Basingstoke.

Barnett S (2002a). Communication with deaf and hard-of-hearing people: A guide for medical education. *Academic Medicine* **77**(7): 694–700.

Barnett S (2002b). Cross-cultural communication with patients who use American Sign Language. *Family Medicine* **34**(5): 376–382.

Bau A (1999). Providing culturally competent services to visually impaired persons. *Journal of Visual Impairment & Blindness (JVIB)* **93**(05).

Beebe SA (1974). Eye contact: A nonverbal determinant of speaker credibility. *Communication Education* **23**(1): 21–25.

Bent T, Bradlow AR, Wright BA (2006). The influence of linguistic experience on the cognitive processing of pitch in speech and nonspeech sounds. *Journal of Experimental Psychology: Human Perception and Performance* **32**(1): 97.

Berger P, Luckmann T (1969). *The Social Construction of Reality: A Treatise in the Sociology of Knowledge*. Penguin Books: St Ives.

Bild (2010). British Institute of Learning Disability Website http://www.bild.org.uk/easy-read/. [Accessed 15/11/10]

Biocca F, Levy MR (2013) (Eds). *Communication in the Age of Virtual Reality*. Lawrence Erlbaum Associates: Hove.

Bischoff R, Reisbig A, Springer P, Schultz S, Robinson W, Olson M (2014). Succeeding in rural mental health practice: Being sensitive to culture by fitting in and collaborating. *Contemporary Family Therapy: An International Journal* **36**(1): 1–16.

Bissell P, May CR, Noyce PR (2004). From compliance to concordance: Barriers to accomplishing a re-framed model of health care interactions. *Social Science & Medicine* **58**(4): 851–862.

Blair J (2011). Care adjustments for people with learning disabilites in hospitals. *Nursing Management* **18**(8): 21–24.

Bourdieu P (1991). *Language and Symbolic Power*. Polity Press: Cambridge, UK.

Bowe H, Martin K (2007). *Communication Across Cultures: Mutual Understanding in a Global World*. Cambridge University Press: Cambridge; New York; Melbourne; Madrid.

Bradbury-Jones C, Sambrook S, Irvine F (2008). Power and empowerment in nursing: A fourth theoretical approach. *Journal of Advanced Nursing* **62**(2): 258–266.

Bradley E, Lofchy J (2005). Learning disability in the accident and emergency department. *Advances in Psychiatric Treatment* **11**(1): 45–57.

Bradshaw J (2013). The use of augmentative and alternative communication apps for the iPad, iPod and iPhone: An overview of recent developments. *Tizard Learning Disability Review* **18**(1): 31–37.

Brumback RA, Staton RD (1983). Learning disability and childhood depression. *American Journal of Orthopsychiatry* **53**(2): 269.

Bryan K, Axelrod L, Maxim J, Bell L, Jordan L (2002). Working with older people with communication difficulties: An evaluation of care worker training. *Aging & mental health* **6**(3): 248–254.

Bull P (1983). *Body Movement and Interpersonal Communication*. John Wiley & Sons Inc: New York.

Bullowa M (1979). *Before Speech: The Beginning of Interpersonal Communication*. Cambridge University Press: London; New York; Melbourne.

Bunning K, Gona JK, Buell S, Newton CR, Hartley S (2013). Investigation of practices to support the complex communication needs of children with hearing impairment and cerebral palsy in a rural district of Kenya: A case series. *International Journal of Language & Communication Disorders* **48**(6): 689–702.

Bunning K, Heath B, Minnion A (2009). Communication and empowerment: A place for rich and multiple media? *Journal of Applied Research in Intellectual Disabilities* **22**(4): 370.

Burns JA, Kintz B (1976). Eye contact while lying during an interview. *Bulletin of the Psychonomic Society* **7**(1): 87–89.

Cain K, Oakhill J (eds) (2007). *Children's Comprehension Problems in Oral and Written Language: A Cognitive Perspective*. Guildford Press: New York.

Callister LC (2003). Cultural influences on pain perceptions and behaviors. *Home Health Care Management & Practice* **15**(3): 207–211.

Callister LC, Luthy KE, Thompson P, Memmott RJ (2009). Ethical reasoning in baccalaureate nursing students. *Nursing ethics* **16**(4): 499–510.

Cameron V (2013). Best practices for stroke patient and family education in the acute care setting: A literature review. *MEDSURG Nursing* **22**(1): 51–55.

Carpiac-Claver ML, Levy-Storms L (2007). In a manner of speaking: Communication between nurse aides and older adults in long-term care settings. *Health communication* **22**(1): 59–67.

Carr SM (2004). A framework for understanding clinical reasoning in community nursing. *Journal of clinical nursing* **13**(7): 850–857.

Cascella PW (2005). Expressive communication strengths of adults with severe to profound intellectual disabilities as reported by group home staff. *Communication Disorders Quarterly* **26**(3): 156.

Chambers S (2003). Use of non-verbal communication skills to improve nursing care. *British Journal of Nursing*. Mark Allen Publishing Limited: London. **12**: 874–879.

Chang M, Hsu L (2007). The perceptions of Taiwanese families who have children with learning disability. *Journal of Clinical Nursing* **16**(12): 2349–2356.

Chant S, Jenkinson T, Randle J, Russell G, Webb C (2002). Communication skills training in healthcare: A review of the literature. *Nurse Education Today* **22**(3): 189–202.

Chen G-M, Starosta WJ (1996a). Intercultural communication competence: A synthesis. *Communication Yearbook* **19**(1): 353–384.

Chen GM, Starosta WJ (1996b). Inter-cultural competence: A synthesis. In: Burleson BR. *Communication Yearbook 19*. Sage: Thousand Oaks CA.

Chomsky N (1965). *Aspects of the Theory of Syntax*. MIT: Massachusetts.

Christine Edwards S (1998). An anthropological interpretation of nurses' and patients' perceptions of the use of space and touch. *Journal of Advanced Nursing* **28**(4): 809–817.

Clarke ME, Pierson W (1999). Management of elder abuse in the emergency department. *Emergency Medicine Clinics of North America* **17**(3): 631–644.

Coleman A, Weir KA, Ware RS, Boyd RN (2013). Relationship between communication skills and gross motor function in preschool-aged children with cerebral palsy. *Archives of Physical Medicine & Rehabilitation* **94**(11): 2210–2217.

Colman RS, Frankel F, Ritvo E, Freeman B (1976). The effects of fluorescent and incandescent illumination upon repetitive behaviors in autistic children. *Journal of Autism and Childhood Schizophrenia* **6**(2): 157–162.

Comas-Diaz L (2012). *Multicultural Care: A Clinician's Guide to Cultural Competence*. American Psychological Association: Washington, DC.

Connection CC (1987). Chinese values and the search for culture- free dimensions of culture. *Journal of Cross Cultural Psychology* **18**(143–164).

Cook, G, Yohannes I, Le Scoullier S, Booy D (2005). Lighting the homes of people who are visually impaired. *International Congress Series*. Elsevier.

Cooke D (1959). *The Language of Music*. Oxford University Press: Oxford.

Cooney C, Howard R, Lawlor B (2006). Abuse of vulnerable people with dementia by their carers: Can we identify those most at risk? *International Journal of Geriatric Psychiatry* **21**(6): 564–571.

Cossins D (2012). Who discovered that the first four notes of Beethoven's 5th Symphony could be used as propaganda 'psych-weapon'? In: *History Extra*, History B [Accessed 21/5/2014].

COT (2015). *College of Occupational Therapists Code of Ethics and Professional Conduct*. London: COT.

Courtis JK (2004). Colour as visual rhetoric in financial reporting. *Accounting Forum*. **28** (3) 265–281.

Croom AM (2012). Aesthetic concepts, perceptual learning, and linguistic enculturation: Considerations from Wittgenstein, language, and music. *Integrative Psychological & Behavioral Science* **46**(1): 90–117.

Crowe MT, O'Malley J (2006). Teaching critical reflection skills for advanced mental health nursing practice: a deconstructive–reconstructive approach. *Journal of Advanced Nursing* **56**(1): 79–87.

Culler J (1976). *Saussure*. Fontana Press: London.

Cumella S, Martin D (2004). Secondary healthcare and learning disability results of consensus development conferences. *Journal of Learning Disabilities* **8**(1): 30–40.

Currie G, Burgess N, Hayton JC (2015). HR practices and knowledge brokering by hybrid middle managers in hospital settings: The influence of professional hierarchy. *Human Resource Management*.

Dahl R (1968). Power. In: Sills DL *International Encyclopaedia of Social Science*, Vol. 12. Cromwell Collier and MacMillan Inc: New York.

Dalke H, Little J, Niemann E, Camgoz N, Steadman G, Hill S, *et al*. (2006). Colour and lighting in hospital design. *Optics & Laser Technology* **38**(4): 343–365.

Dana RH (2011). Human science and multicultural assessment practice. *Cultural Competence in Assessment, Diagnosis, and Intervention with Ethnic Minorities: Some Perspectives from Psychology, Social Work, and Education*: 97.

Dancer S (2010). Pants, policies and paranoia *Journal of Hospital Infection* **74**(1): 10–15.

Danielsson H, Ronnberg J, Andersson J (2006). What am I doing in Timbuktu: Person-environment picture recognition for persons with intellectual disability. *Journal of Intellectual Disability Research* **50**(Part 2): 127–138.

Danziger K (1976). *Interpersonal Communication*. Pergamon Press Inc.: New York; Toronto; Oxford; Sydney; Paris.

Darwin C, Bynum WF (2009). *The Origin of Species by Means of Natural Selection: Or, the Preservation of Favored Races in the Struggle for Life*. AL Burt.

Davis MH (1983). Measuring individual differences in empathy: Evidence for a multidimensional approach. *Journal of personality and social psychology* **44**(1): 113.

Davis TR (1984). The influence of the physical environment in offices. *Academy of Management Review* **9**(2): 271–283.

de Vries K (2013). Communicating with older people with dementia. *Nursing Older People* **25**(4): 30–38.

Department of Health (2007). *Independence, Choice and Risk: A Guide to Best Practice in Supported Decision Making*. Gateway number 7733. London.

Department of Health (2011). *No Health without Mental Health*, Health DoH. London: DoH.

Department of Health (2009). *Valuing People Now: A New Three Year Strategy for People with Learning Disabilities*. London: HMSO.

Department of Health (2005). *Mental Capacity Act*, DoH. London: HMSO.

Department of Health (2006). *Our Health, Our Care, Our Say: A New Direction for Community Services*. London: The Stationery Office.

Department of Health (2012). Transforming Care: A national response to Winterbourne View Hospital. *Department of Health Review: Final Report*.

Detaille SI, Haafkens JA, van Dijk FJH (2003). What employees with rheumatoid arthritis, diabetes mellitus and hearing loss need to cope at work. *Scandinavian Journal of Work, Environment & Health* **29**(2): 134–142.

Devito JA (1997). *Human Communication (Seventh Edition)*. Longman: New York.

DHHS U (2014). *National Plan to Address Alzheimer's Disease: 2014 Update*. US: US Department of Health and Human Services.

Diehl J, Bennetto L, Watson D, Gunlogson C, McDonough J (2008). Resolving ambiguity: A psycholinguistic approach to understanding prosody processing in high-functioning autism. *Brain and Language* **106**: 144–152.

Dijkstra K, Pieterse ME, Pruyn ATH (2008). Individual differences in reactions towards color in simulated healthcare environments: The role of stimulus screening ability. *Journal of environmental psychology* **28**(3): 268–277.

Dobson S, Upadhyaya S, Conyers I, Raghavan R (2002). Touch in the care of people with profound and complex needs: a review of the literature. *Journal of Learning Disabilities (14690047)* **6**(4): 351–362.

Dougherty L, Lister S (2011). *The Royal Marsden Hospital Manual of Clinical Nursing Procedures*. edn. John Wiley & Sons.

Drew T, Võ ML-H, Wolfe JM (2013). The invisible gorilla strikes again: sustained inattentional blindness in expert observers. *Psychological Science* **24**(9): 1848–1853.

Dunn MC, Clare IC, Holland AJ (2008). To empower or to protect? Constructing the 'vulnerable adult' in English law and public policy. *Legal Studies* **28**(2): 234–253.

Edelstein AS, Ito Y, Kepplinger HM (1989). *Communication and Culture: A Comparative Approach*. Longman Inc: White Plains, NY.

Edwards J, Jackson HJ, Pattison PE (2002). Emotion recognition via facial expression and affective prosody in schizophrenia: A methodological review. *Clinical Psychology Review* **22**(6): 789–832.

Eggenberger E, Heimerl K, Bennett MI (2013). Communication skills training in dementia care: A systematic review of effectiveness, training content, and didactic methods in different care settings. *International Psychogeriatrics/IPA* **25**(3): 345–358.

Eigsti I, Marchena A, Schuh J, Kelly E (2011). Language acquisition in autistic spectrum disorders: A developmental review. *Research in Autism Spectrum Disorders* **5**: 681–691.

Ekman P (1976). Movements with precise meanings. *Journal of Communication* **26**(3): 14–26.

Ekman P, Friesen WV, Ellsworth P (2013). *Emotion in the Human Face: Guidelines for Research and an Integration of Findings*. Permagon Press: New York; Ontario; Oxford; Sydney.

Embregts P, van Nieuwenhuijzen M (2009). Social information processing in boys with autistic spectrum disorder and mild to borderline intellectual disabilities. *Journal Of Intellectual Disability Research* **53**(11): 922.

Fărcaş A, Roth M (2004). Preschool And primary school teachers' role in detecting and reporting child abuse and neglect cases. *Educaţia-Plus Journal Plus Education*: 9.

Farroni T, Csibra G, Simion F, Johnson MH (2002). Eye contact detection in humans from birth. *Proceedings of the National Academy of Sciences* **99**(14): 9602–9605.

Feil N (2014). Validation therapy with late-onset dementia populations. *Caregiving in Dementia: Research and Applications*: 199–218.

Fellinger J, Holzinger D, Pollard R (2012). Mental health of deaf people. *The Lancet* **379**(9820): 1037–1044.

Finlay WML, Antaki C, Walton C (2007). On not being noticed: Intellectual disabilities and the nonvocal register. *Intellectual and Developmental Disabilities* **45**(4): 227–245.

Finlay WML, Antaki C, Walton C (2008a). Saying no to the staff: An analysis of refusals in a home for people with severe communication difficulties. *Sociology of Health & Illness* **30**(1): 55–75.

Finlay WML, Antaki C, Walton C, Stribling P (2008b). The dilemma for staff in 'playing a game' with a person with profound intellectual disabilities: Empowerment, inclusion and competence in interactional practice. *Sociology of Health & Illness* **30**(4): 531–549.

Finlay WML, Walton C, Antaki C (2008c). Promoting choice and control in residential services for people with learning disabilities. *Disability & Society* **23**(4): 349–360.

Fisher JD, Rytting M, Heslin R (1976). Hands touching hands: Affective and evaluative effects of an interpersonal touch. *Sociometry*: 416–421.

Flynn M (2012). Winterbourne View Hospital: A Serious Case Review, Board SGSA (ed). South Gloucestershire.

Flynn M, Hollins S (2013). Acting on the lessons of Winterbourne View Hospital. *BMJ* **346**: 18.

Foucault M (1965). *History of Madness*. Tavistock Publications/Routledge: London; New York.

Francis R (2013). *Report of the Mid Staffordshire NHS Foundation Trust Public Inquiry: Executive Summary*. vol. 947. The Stationery Office.

Friere P (1986). *Pedagagy of the Oppressed*. Penguin: Harmondsworth.

Galasiński D, Ziółkowska J (2007). Gender and the gynecological examination Women's identities in doctors' narratives. *Qualitative Health Research* **17**(4): 477–488.

Gazzaniga MS, Ivry RB, Mangun GR (2002). *Cognitive Neuroscience: The Biology of the Mind (Second Edition)*. W.W. Norton: New York; London.

Geissmann T (2000). Gibbon songs and human music from an evolutionary perspective. *The Origins of Music*: 103–123.

Gibbs SM, Brown MJ, Muir WJ (2008). The experiences of adults with intellectual disabilities and their carers in general hospitals: A focus group study. *Journal of Intellectual Disability Research* **52**(12): 1061–1077.

Gilbert T, Cochrane A, Greenwell S (2003). Professional discourse and service cultures: An organisational typology developed from health and welfare services for people with learning disabilities. *International Journal of Nursing Studies* **40**(7): 781.

Goffman E (1968). *Asylums: Essays on the Social Situation of Mental Patients and Other Inmates*. AldineTransaction.

Goffman E (1981). *Forms of Talk*. University of Pennsylvania Press: Philadelphia.

Goffman E (1967). *Interaction Ritual*. Doubleday Anchor: New York.

Goffman E (1961). *On the Characteristics of Total Institutions*. Penguin: London; New York; Victoria.

Goffman E (1959). *The Presentation of Self in Everyday Life*. Penguin Books: London; New York; Victoria.

Goffman E (1963). *Stigma: Notes on the Management of Spoiled Identity*. Penguin Books: London; New York; Victoria.

Goldbart J, Caton S (2010). *Communication and People with the Most Complex Needs: What Works and Why this is Essential*. Mencap: London.

Goodey CF (2004). 'Foolishness' in early modern medicine and the concept of intellectual disability. *Medical History* **48**(3): 289–310.

Goodey CF (2011). *A History of Intelligence and 'Intellectual Disability': The Shaping of Psychology in Early Modern Europe*. Ashgate Publishing Ltd: Farnham, Surrey; Burlington, VT.

Gordon MM, Hampson R, Capell H, Madhok R (2002). Illiteracy in rheumatoid arthritis patients as determined by the Rapid Estimate of Adult Literacy in Medicine (REALM) score. *Rheumatology* **41**(7): 750–754.

Graham J (2004). Communicating with the uncommunicative: Music therapy with pre-verbal adults. *British Journal of Learning Disabilities* **32**(1): 24–29.

Gray C, Murphey J, Cox S (2007). *How Talking Mats Can Help People with Dementia to Communicate*. Joseph Rowntree Foundation: York.

Gumperz JJ (1978). The conversational analysis of interethnic communication. *Interethnic Communication*: 13–31.

Hall E (2004). Social geographies of learning disability: Narratives of exclusion and inclusion. *Area* **36**(3): 298–306.

Hall ET (1977). *Beyond Culture*. Doubleday: Garden City, NY.

Hall ET (1966). *The Hidden Dimension*. Doubleday: Garden City, NY.

Hall ET (1959). *The Silent Language*. Anchor Books: New York.

Hardy K, O'Brien S, Furlong N (2001). Quality improvement report: Information given to patients before appointments and its effect on non-attendance rate. *BMJ: British Medical Journal* **323**(7324): 1298.

Hargie O, Marshall P (1997). Interpersonal communication: A theoretical framework. *The Handbook of Communication Skills* **2**: 29–63.

Harris J (1995). Boiled eggs and baked beans – a personal account of a hearing researcher's journey through deaf culture. *Disability & Society* **10**(3): 295–308.

Hatton N (2009). The labelling effect: drama, mental health and learning disability. *Research in Drama Education* **14**(1): 91–95.

Haugaard M (ed) (2002). *Power: A Reader*. Manchester University Press: Manchester; New York.

Hemsley B, Balandin S, Worrall L (2011). The 'Big 5' and beyond: Nurses, paid carers, and adults with developmental disability discuss communication needs in hospital. *Applied Nursing Research* **24**(4): e51–58.

Hemsley B, Sigafoos J, Balandin S, Forbes R, Taylor C, Green VA, *et al.* (2001). Nursing the patient with severe communication impairment. *Journal of Advanced Nursing* **35**(6): 827–835.

Hepworth D, Rooney R, Rooney GD, Strom-Gottfried K, Larsen JA (2009). *Direct Social Work Practice: Theory and Skills (Eighth Edition)*. Cengage Learning. Brooks /Cole: Belmont CA.

Heslop P, Blair P, Fleming P, Hoghton M, Marriott A, Russ L (2013). Confidential inquiry into premature deaths of people with learning disabilities (CIPOLD). *Bristol: Norah Fry Research Centre*.

Higgs J, Jones MA, Loftus S, Christensen N (2008). *Clinical Reasoning in the Health Professions (Third Edition)*. Elsevier Limited: Amsterdam; Boston; Heidelberg; London.

Hill G, Thompson G, Willis S, Hodgson D (2014). Embracing service user involvement in radiotherapy education: A discussion paper. *Radiography* **20**(1): 82–86.

Hirschi T (1975). Labelling theory and juvenile delinquency: An assessment of the evidence. *The Labeling of Deviance: Evaluating a Perspective*. New York: Wiley: 181–203.

Hofstede G (1994). Business cultures. *UNESCO Courier* **47**(4): 12–16.

Hofstede G (2001). *Culture's Consequences: Comparing Values, Behaviours, Institutions and Organisations across Nations (Second Edition)*. Sage: Thousand Oaks, CA.

Hofstede G (1997). *Cultures and Organisations: Software of the Mind (Revised Edition)*. McGraw-Hill: New York.

Hofstede G, Bond MH (1984). Hofstede's cultural dimensions: An independent valida-tion using Rokeach's value survey. *Journal of Cross Cultural Psychology* **15**: 417–433.

Horner-Johnson W, Keys C, Henry D, Yamaki K, Oi F, Watanabe K, *et al.* (2002). Attitudes of Japanese students toward people with intellectual disability. *Journal Of Intellectual Disability Research* **46**(5): 365.

Horsburgh M, Perkins R, Coyle B, Degeling P (2006). The professional subcultures of students entering medicine, nursing and pharmacy programmes. *Journal of interprofessional care* **20**(4): 425–431.

Hsu FLK (1969). *The Study of Literate Civilisations.* Holt, Rhinehart and Winston: New York.

Hubert J (2006). Family carers' views of services for people with learning disabilities from black and minority ethnic groups: A qualitative study of 30 families in a south London borough. *Disability & Society* **21**(3): 259–272.

Huss M, Verney JP, Fosker T, Mead N, Goswami U (2011). Music, rhythm, rise time perception and developmental dyslexia: Perception of musical meter predicts reading and phonology. *Cortex: A Journal Devoted to the Study of the Nervous System & Behavior* **47**(6): 674–689.

Hymes D (2005). Models of the interaction of language and social life: Towards a descriptive theory. In: Kiesling F, Bratt-Paulston C (eds) *Intercultural Discourse and Communication: The Essential Readings,* Malden, USA; Oxford, UK: Blackwell Publishing.

Iacono T, Davis R (2003). The experiences of people with developmental disabil-ity in emergency departments and hospital wards. *Research in Developmental Disabilities* **24**(4): 247–264.

Inalhan G, Gorgievski MJ, van der Voordt TJ, van Herpen SG, van Akkeren S (2010). After the fire: New ways of working in an academic setting. *Facilities* **28**(3/4): 206–224.

Ingold T (2004). Culture on the ground the world perceived through the feet. *Journal of Material Culture* **9**(3): 315–340.

Iwakuma M (2002). The body as embodiment: An investigation of the body by Merleau-Ponty. *Disability, Postmodernity, Embodying Disability Theory*: 76–87.

Izard CE (1994). Innate and universal facial expressions: Evidence from developmen-tal and cross-cultural research. *Psychological Bulletin* **115**(2): 288–299.

Jandt FE (2007). *An Introduction to Intercultural Communication.* Sage Publications Inc: Thousand Oaks, CA; London; Delhi.

Jane Ward D (2007). Hand adornment and infection control. *British Journal Of Nursing* **16**(11): 654–656.

John'a S (1991). Music structure and emotional response: Some empirical findings. *Psychology of Music* **991**(9): L120.

John J (1996). A dramaturgical view of the health care service encounter: cultural value-based impression management guidelines for medical professional behav-iour. *European Journal of Marketing* **30**(9): 60–74.

Johnson H, Douglas J, Bigby C, Iacono T (2010). The pearl in the middle: A case study of social interactions in an individual with a severe intellectual disability. *Journal of Intellectual & Developmental Disability* **35**(3): 175–186.

Jones R, Quigney C, Huws J (2003). First-hand accounts of sensory perceptual experiences in autism: A qualitative analysis. *Journal of Intellectual and Developmental Disability* **28**(2): 112–121.

Juslin PN, Sloboda JA (2010). *Handbook of Music and Emotion: Theory, Research, Applications*. Oxford University Press: Oxford.

Kacperek L (1997). Clinical. Non-verbal communication: The importance of listening. *British Journal of Nursing (BJN)* **6**(5): 275–279.

Kastner MP, Crowder RG (1990). Perceptions of the major minor distinction: IV emotional connotations in young children. *Music Perception* **8**: 189 - 202.

Keane J, Calder AJ, Hodges JR, Young AW (2002). Face and emotion processing in frontal variant frontotemporal dementia. *Neuropsychologia* **40**(6): 655–665.

Kennedy K, Mercer RE (2002). Planning animation cinematography and shot structure to communicate theme and mood. *Proceedings of the 2nd International Symposium on Smart Graphics*. ACM. pp. 1–8.

Kidd J (2010). Cultural boundary surfing in mental health nursing: A creative narration. *Contemporary Nurse: A Journal for the Australian Nursing Profession* **34**(2): 277–288.

Kielhofner G (2008). *Model of Human Occupation: Theory and Application (Fourth Edition)*. Lippincott, Williams and Wilkins: Baltimore; Philadelphia.

Kiesling SF (2005). Norms of sociocultural meaning in language. In: Kiesling SF, Bratt-Paulston C (eds). *Intercultural Discourse and Communication: The Essential Readings*, edn. Malden, USA; Oxford; Victoria: Blackwell Publishing Ltd.

Kington J, Jones L, Watt A, Hopkin E, Williams J (2000). Impaired eye expression recognition in schizophrenia. *Journal of Psychiatric Research* **34**(4): 341–347.

Knapp M, Hall J, Horgan T (2013). *Nonverbal Communication in Human Interaction*. Cengage Learning/Wadsworth: Australia; Brazil; Japan; Korea; United Kingdom.

Koolhof M, Fenton J, Richardson AE, Richardson E (2013). *When Mummy Shouts: A Children's Book about Feeling Safe and Staying with Family*. The Salvation Army and Communities for Children South East Tasmania.

Korduba OM (1975). Duplicated rhythmic patterns between deaf and normal hearing children. *Journal of Music Therapy* **12**(3): 136–146.

Kratus J (1993). A developmental study of children's interpretation of emotion in music. *Psychology of Music* **21**: 3–19.

Kress G (2009). *Multimodality: A Social Semiotic Approach to Contemporary Communication*. Routledge, Taylor and Francis Group: London; New York.

Kruijver IPM, Kerkstra A, Kerssens JJ, Holtkamp CCM, Bensing JM, Hbm (2001). Communication between nurses and simulated patients with cancer: Evaluation of a communication training programme... including commentary by Heaven C and Payne S. *European Journal of Oncology Nursing* **5**(3): 140–153.

Kurtz SM, Silverman DJ, Draper J, van Dalen J, Platt FW (2005). *Teaching and Learning Communication Skills in Medicine*. Radcliffe Publishers: Oxford.

Labov W (1972). *Language in the Inner City: Studies in the Black English Vernacular*. University of Pennsylvania Press: Pennsylvania.

Lachetta R, Tacke D, Doerscheln I, Schulz M (2011). The experiences of people with learning disability in acute hospitals – a systematic literature review [German]. *Pflegewissenschaft* **13**(3): 139–148.

Laird SE (2008). *Anti-oppressive Social Work: A Guide for Developing Cultural Competence.* Sage Publications: Thousand Oaks, CA.

Lancioni GE, Bosco A, Belardinelli MO, Singh NN, O'Reilly MF, Sigafoos J (2010). An overview of intervention options for promoting adaptive behavior of persons with acquired brain injury and minimally conscious state. *Research in Developmental Disabilities* **31**(6): 1121–1134.

Lancioni GE, Singh NN, O'Reilly MF, Sigafoos J, Belardinelli MO, Buonocunto F, *et al.* (2012). Promoting adaptive behavior in persons with acquired brain injury, extensive motor and communication disabilities, and consciousness disorders. *Research In Developmental Disabilities* **33**(6): 1964–1974.

Laverack G (2005). *Public Health: Power, Empowerment and Professional Practice.* Palgrave Macmillan: Basingstoke, UK; New York, USA.

Leathers D, Eaves M (2008). *Successful Nonverbal Communication (4th).* Allyn and Bacon: Boston.

Leitman DI, Foxe JJ, Butler PD, Saperstein A, Revheim N, Javitt DC (2005). Sensory contributions to impaired prosodic processing in schizophrenia. *Biological Psychiatry* **58**(1): 56–61.

Lernihan E, Sweeney J (2010). Measuring levels of burnout among care workers. *Learning Disability Practice* **13**(8): 27–33.

Leucht S, Burkard T, Henderson J, Maj M, Sartorius N (2007). Physical illness and schizophrenia: A review of the literature. *Acta Psychiatrica Scandinavica* **116**(5): 317–333.

Lewin S, Skea Z, Entwistle VA, Zwarenstein M, Dick J (2001). Interventions for providers to promote a patient-centred approach in clinical consultations. *Cochrane Database of Systematic Reviews* (4): 10.

Lieu CC-h, Sadler GR, Fullerton JT, Stohlmann PD (2007). Communication strategies for nurses interacting with patients who are deaf. *Dermatology Nursing* **19**(6): 541.

Liew S-M, Tong SF, Lee VKM, Ng CJ, Leong KC, Teng CL (2009). Text messaging reminders to reduce non-attendance in chronic disease follow-up: A clinical trial. *British Journal of General Practice* **59**(569): 916–920.

Lim HA (2010). Effect of 'Developmental speech and language training through music' on speech production in children with autism spectrum disorder. *Journal of Music Therapy* **47**(1): 2–26.

Livingston G, Johnston K, Katona C, Paton J, Lyketsos CG, Psychiatry OATFotWFoB (2014). Systematic review of psychological approaches to the management of neuropsychiatric symptoms of dementia. *American Journal of Psychiatry.*

Lomas KJ, Giridharan R (2012). Thermal comfort standards, measured internal temperatures and thermal resilience to climate change of free-running buildings: A case-study of hospital wards. *Building and Environment* **55**: 57–72.

Lukes S (1974). *Power: A Radical View.* Palgrave Macmillan: London.

Lyman SM, Scott MB (1967). Territoriality: A neglected sociological dimension. *Social Problems* **15**(2): 236–249.

Mackenzie L (2007). 'Does this look like a disability to you' stories as a tool for the creation of an alternative identity in a music-based learning community. *Storytelling, Self, Society* **3**(2): 115–134.

Maginess T (2010). Medium as message: making an 'emancipating' film on mental health and distress. *Educational Action Research* **18**(4): 497–515.

Marsh PE (1988). *Eye to Eye: how People Interact.* Salem House Publishers: Toppsfield, MA.

Martens MA, Jungers MK, Steele AL (2011). Effect of musical experience on verbal memory in Williams syndrome: Evidence from a novel word learning task. *Neuropsychologia* **49**(11): 3093–3102.

Mashal N, Kasirer A (2012). Principal component analysis study of visual and verbal metaphoric comprehension in children with autism and learning disabilities. *Research In Developmental Disabilities* **33**(1): 274–282.

Mast MS (2007). On the importance of nonverbal communication in the physician–patient interaction. *Patient Education and Counseling* **67**(3): 315–318.

Matsumoto D (1989). Cultural influences on the perception of emotion. *Journal of Cross-Cultural Psychology* **20**(1): 92–105.

Mattingly C, Hayes Fleming M (1994). *Clincial Reasoning: Forms of Inquiry in a Therapeutic Practice.* FA Davis Company: Philadelphia.

McCann J, Peppe S, Gibbon FE, O'Hare A, Rutherford M (2007). Prosody and its relationship to language in school-aged children with high-functioning autism. *International Journal of Language and Communication Disorders* **42**: 682–702.

McCann K, McKenna HP (1993). An examination of touch between nurses and elderly patients in a continuing care setting in Northern Ireland. *Journal of Advanced Nursing* **18**(5): 838–846.

McCarthy V, Holbrook Freeman L (2008). A Multidisciplinary Concept of Empowerment: Implications for Nursing. *Journal of Theory Construction and Testing* **12**(2): 68.

McCloskey RM (2004). Caring for patients with dementia in an acute care environ-ment. *Geriatric Nursing* **25**(3): 139–144.

McConkey R, Morris I, Purcell M (1999). Communications between staff and adults with intellectual disabilities in naturally occurring settings. *Journal of Intellectual Disability Research* **43**(3): 194–205.

McDermott GL, McDonnell AM (2014). Acquired brain injury services in the Republic of Ireland: Experiences and perceptions of families and professionals. *Brain Injury* **28**(1): 81–91.

McLaughlin H (2009). What's in a name: 'client','patient','customer','consumer', 'expert by experience','service user' – what's next? *British Journal of Social Work* **39**(6): 1101–1117.

Mehrabian A (1969). Significance of posture and position in the communication of attitude and status relationships. *Psychological Bulletin* **71**(5): 359.

Mehrabian A (1971). *Silent Messages.* Wadsworth: Oxford, UK.

Mencap (2013). *1200 Avoidable Deaths.* Mencap: London.

Mencap (2006). *Death by Indifference.* Mencap: London.

Mencap (nd). Make it Clear. www.Mencap.org [Accessed 15/3/14].

Michael J, Richardson A (2008). *Healthcare for All: The Independent Inquiry into Access to Healthcare for People with Learning Disabilities.* Department of Health: London.

Millward LJ, Haslam SA, Postmes T (2007). Putting employees in their place: The impact of hot desking on organizational and team identification. *Organization Science* **18**(4): 547–559.

Moog H (1976). The musical experience of the pre-school child. *Psychology of Music* 4(2): 38–45.

Moore BC (2008). The role of temporal fine structure processing in pitch perception, masking, and speech perception for normal-hearing and hearing-impaired people. *Journal of the Association for Research in Otolaryngology* **9**(4): 399–406.

Moyle W, Olorenshaw R, Wallis M, Borbasi S (2008). Best practice for the management of older people with dementia in the acute care setting: A review of the literature. *International Journal of Older People Nursing* **3**(2): 121–130.

Narey M (2014). *Making the Education of Social Workers Consistently Effective*: Report of Sir Martin Narey's independent review of the education of children's social workers (2014).

Neugebauer R (1996). Mental handicap in medieval and early modern England: Criteria, measurement and care. In: *From Idiocy to Mental Deficiency*, Digby A, Wright D (eds). Routledge: London; New York.

Neuliep JW (2009). *Intercultural Communication: A Contextual Approach.* edn. SAGE Publications Inc: Thousand Oaks, CA; New Delhi; London.

NHS (2015a). NHS Vision and Values. www.nhs [Accessed 11/6/15].

NHS (2015b). Values Based Recruitment. www.nhs [Accessed 11/6/15].

Nimmon LE (2007). ESL-speaking immigrant women's disillusions: Voices of health care in Canada: An ethnodrama. *Health Care for Women International* **28**(4): 381–396.

Nind M, Flewitt R, Payler J (2010). The social experience of early childhood for children with learning disabilities: Inclusion, competence and agency. *British Journal of Sociology of Education* **31**(6): 653–670.

Nursing, Midwifery C (2008). *The Code: Standards of Conduct, Performance and Ethics for Nurses and Midwives.* NMC: London.

O'Leary KD, Rosenbaum A, Hughes PC (1978). Fluorescent lighting: A purported source of hyperactive behavior. *Journal of Abnormal Child Psychology* **6**(3): 285–289.

Ochs E (1993). Constructing social identity: A language socialization perspective. *Research on language and Social Interaction* **26**(3): 287–306.

Ong LM, Visser MR, Lammes FB, De Haes JC (2000). Doctor–patient communication and cancer patients' quality of life and satisfaction. *Patient Education and Counseling* **41**(2): 145–156.

Osgood CE (1970). Speculation on the structure of interpersonal intentions. *Behavioral Science* **15**(3): 237–254.

Oxenham AJ (2008). Pitch perception and auditory stream segregation: Implications for hearing loss and cochlear implants. *Trends in Amplification* **12**(4): 316–331.

Ozbič M, Filipčič T (2010). Complex imitation of gestures in school-aged children with learning difficulties. *Imitiranje Složenih Pokreta Kod Školske Djece S Poteškoćama U Učenju.* **42**(1): 44–55.

Park S-H, Ku J, Kim J-J, Jang HJ, Kim SY, Kim SH, *et al.* (2009). Increased personal space of patients with schizophrenia in a virtual social environment. *Psychiatry Research* **169**(3): 197–202.

Parsons T (1951). *The Social System.* Appleton and Lange: Norwalk, CT.

Passalacqua SA, Harwood J (2012). VIPS communication skills training for paraprofessional dementia caregivers: An intervention to increase person-centered dementia care. *Clinical Gerontologist* **35**(5): 425–445.

Pattison JE (1973). Effects of touch on self-exploration and the therapeutic relationship. *Journal of Consulting and Clinical Psychology* **40**(2): 170.

Pearson A, Baker H, Walsh K, Fitzgerald M (2001). Contemporary nurses' uniforms – history and traditions. *Journal of Nursing Management* **9**(3): 147–152.

Perry J, Watkins M, Gilbert A, Rawlinson J (2013). A systematic review of the evidence on service user involvement in interpersonal skills training of mental health students. *Journal of Psychiatric & Mental Health Nursing* **20**(6): 525–540.

Phillips J (2005). Knowledge is power: Using nursing information management and leadership interventions to improve services to patients, clients and users. *Journal of Nursing Management* **13**(6): 524–536.

Philpsen G (1975). Speaking like a man in 'Teamsterville': Culture patterns of role enactment in an urban neighbourhood. *Quarterly Journal of Speech* **62**: 15–25.

Potts P (2000). Concrete representations of a social category: Consolidating and transforming public institutions for people classified as 'defective'. In: *Crossing Boundaries: Change and Continuity in the History of Learning Disability*, Brigham L, Atkinson D, Jackson M, Rolph S, Walmsley J (eds). BILD Publications: Kidderminster.

Pratt MG, Rafaeli A (1997). Organizational dress as a symbol of multilayered social identities. *Academy of Management Journal* **40**(4): 862–898.

Price B (2013). Countering the stereotype of the unpopular patient. *Nursing Older People* **25**(6): 27–35.

Raghavan R (2009). Improving access to services for minority ethnic communities. *Learning Disability Practice* **12**(7): 14–18.

Ragneskog H, Gerdner LA, Josefsson K, Kihlgren M (1998). Probable reasons for expressed agitation in persons with dementia. *Clinical Nursing Research* **7**(2): 189–206.

Ramcharan P (1997). *Empowerment in Everyday Life: Learning Disability.* Jessica Kingsley Publications: London.

Ramcharan P, Grant G (2001). Views and expereinces of people with intellectual disabilities and their families (1) The user perspective. *Journal of Applied Research in Intellectual Disabilities* **14**(Journal Article): 348–353.

Reamer FG (2013). *Social Work Values and Ethics.* Columbia University Press: Columbia.

Regnard C, Reynolds J, Watson B, Matthews D, Gibson L, Clarke C (2007). Understanding distress in people with severe communication difficulties: developing and assessing the Disability Distress Assessment Tool (DisDAT). *Journal of Intellectual Disability Research* **51**(Part 4): 277–292.

Rogers J (2012). Anti-oppressive social work research: Reflections on power in the creation of knowledge. *Social Work Education* **31**(7): 866–879.

Roter D, Larson S (2002). The Roter interaction analysis system (RIAS): Utility and flexibility for analysis of medical interactions. *Patient Education and Counseling* **46**(4): 243–251.

Rowe MB (1986). Wait time: Slowing down may be a way of speeding up! *Journal of Teacher Education* **37**(1): 43–50.

Sack RD (1986). *Human Territoriality: Its Theory and History*. vol. 7. CUP Archive.

Samovar LA, Porter RE (2004). *Communication between Cultures (5th Edition)*. Wadsworth: Belmont CA.

Sargent J, Clarke M, Price K, Griffiths T, Swettenham J (2013). Use of eye-pointing by children with cerebral palsy: what are we looking at? *International Journal of Language & Communication Disorders* **48**(5): 477–485.

Sasso L, Stievano A, Jurado MG, Rocco G (2008). Code of ethics and conduct for European nursing. *Nursing Ethics* **15**(6): 821–836.

Schaaf RC, Miller LJ (2005). Occupational therapy using a sensory integrative approach for children with developmental disabilities. *Mental Retardation and Developmental Disabilities Research Reviews* **11**(2): 143–148.

Scheckel M, Hedrick-Erickson J (2009). Decentering resources: A phenomenological study of interpretive pedagogies in patient education. *Journal of Professional Nursing* **25**(1): 57–64.

Scheff TJ (1974). The labelling theory of mental illness. *American Sociological Review*: 444–452.

Schein EH (2010). *Organisational Culture and Leadership (Fourth Edition)*. John Wiley and Sons: San Francisco.

Scollon R, Scollon-Wong S, Jones HJ (2012). *Intercultural Communication: A Discourse Approach (Third Edition)*. Wiley-Blackwell: Malden, MA; Oxford; Chichester.

Seabury BA (1971). Arrangement of physical space in social work settings. *Social Work*: 43–49.

Segal JZ (2007). 'Compliance' to 'concordance': A critical view. *Journal of Medical Humanities* **28**(2): 81–96.

Senju A, Johnson MH (2009). Atypical eye contact in autism: Models, mechanisms and development. *Neuroscience & Biobehavioral Reviews* **33**(8): 1204–1214.

Shattell M (2004). Nurse–patient interaction: A review of the literature. *Journal of Clinical Nursing* **13**(6): 714–722.

Sheedy M (2013). *Core Themes in Social Work Power, Poverty, Politics and Values*. Open University Press: Maidenhead.

Shome R (1996). Postcolonial interventions in the rhetorical canon: An 'other' view. *Communication Theory* **6**(1): 40–59.

Silverman J, Kurtz SM, Draper J, van Dalen J, Platt FW (1998). Skills for communicating with patients. CRC Press, Taylor Francis Group, Boca Ranton, London, New York.

Simmons P, Hawley CJ, Gale TM, Sivakumaran T (2010). Service user, patient, client, user or survivor: Describing recipients of mental health services. *The Psychiatrist* **34**(1): 20–23.

Simons DJ, Chabris DF (1999). Gorillas in our midst: Sustained inattentional blindness for dynamic events. *Perception* **28**: 1059–1074.

Sloboda JA, Juslin PN (2001). Psychological perspectives on music and emotion.

Smith H (1981). Territorial spacing on a beach revisited: A cross-national exploration. *Social Psychology Quarterly*: 132–137.

Snyder J (2012). How does bullying relate to elder abuse. *Temp. Pol. & Civ. Rts. L. Rev.* **22**: 386.

Sowney M, Barr O (2007). The challenges for nurses communicating with and gaining valid consent from adults with intellectual disabilities within the accident and emergency care service. *Journal Of Clinical Nursing* **16**(9): 1678–1686.

Sprengelmeyer R, Young A, Mahn K, Schroeder U, Woitalla D, Büttner T, *et al.* (2003). Facial expression recognition in people with medicated and unmedicated Parkinson's disease. *Neuropsychologia* **41**(8): 1047–1057.

Stasolla F, Caffò AO, Picucci L, Bosco A (2013). Assistive technology for promoting choice behaviors in three children with cerebral palsy and severe communication impairments. *Research In Developmental Disabilities* **34**(9): 2694–2700.

Stephenson J, Dowrick M (2005). Parents' perspectives on the communication skills of their children with severe disabilities. *Journal of Intellectual & Developmental Disability* **30**(2): 75–85.

Stephenson J, Linfoot K (1996). Pictures as communication symbols for students with severe intellectual disability. *AAC: Augmentative & Alternative Communication* **12**(4): 244–255.

Stevens M, Glendinning C, Jacobs S, Moran N, Challis D, Manthorpe J, *et al.* (2011). Assessing the role of increasing choice in English social care services. *Journal of Social Policy* **40**(2): 257–274.

Stewart M, Brown JB, Boon H, Galajda J, Meredith L, Sangster M (1999). Evidence on patient-doctor communication. *Cancer Prevention & Control* **3**(1): 25–30.

Stoner JB, Beck AR, Bock SJ, Hickey K, Kosuwan K, Thompson JR (2006). The effectiveness of the picture exchange communication system with nonspeaking adults. *Remedial & Special Education* **27**(3): 154–165.

Susan D, Louisa C, Ian C, Shripati U, Raghu R (2004). Learning about touch: An exploratory study to identify the learning needs of staff supporting people with complex needs. *Journal of Learning Disabilities (14690047)* **8**(2): 113–129.

Sweeting H, West P (2001). Being different: Correlates of the experience of teasing and bullying at age 11. *Research Papers in Education* **16**(3): 225–246.

Tager-Flusberg H (1985). Basic level and superordinate level categorization by autistic, mentally retarted and normal children. *Journal of Experiemental Child Psychology* **40**: 450–469.

Tager-Flusberg H, Calkins S (1990). Does imitation facilitate the acquisition of grammar? Evidence from a study of autistic, Down's syndrome and normal children. *Journal Of Child Language* **17**(3): 591–606.

Tager-Flusberg H, Rogers S, Cooper J, Landa R, Lord C, Paul R, *et al.* (2009). Defining spoken language benchmarks and selecting measures of expressive language development for young children with autism spectrum disorders. *Journal of Speech, Language & Hearing Research* **52**(3): 643–652.

Tannen D (2005). New York Jewish conversational style. In: Kiesling SF, Bratt-Paulston C (eds). *Intercultural Discourse and Communication*. Blackwell Publishing: Malden, MA; Oxford; Victoria.

Tate JA, Seaman JB, Happ MB (2012). Overcoming barriers to pain assessment: Communicating pain information with intubated older adults. *Geriatric Nursing* **33**(4): 310.

Taylor Gooby P (2008a). Assumptive worlds and images of agency: Academic social policy in the twenty-first century? *Social Policy and Society* **7**(3): 269–280; 269.

Taylor Gooby P (2008b). Choice and values: Individualised rational action and social goals. *Journal of Social Policy* **37**(2): 167–185.

Thomas B, Courtenay K, Hassiotis A, Strydom A, Rantell K (2014). Standardised patients with intellectual disabilities in training tomorrow's doctors. *Psychiatric Bulletin* **38**(3): 132–136.

Thompson N (2015). *Understanding Social Work: Preparing for Practice*. Palgrave Macmillan: London.

Thurman S, Jones J, Tarleton B (2005). Without words – meaningful information for people with high individual communication needs. *British Journal of Learning Disabilities* **33**(2): 83–89.

Timmons S, East L (2011). Uniforms, status and professional boundaries in hospital. *Sociology of Health & Illness* **33**(7): 1035–1049.

Togher L (2013). Improving communication for people with brain Injury in the 21st century: The value of collaboration. *Brain Impairment* **14**(1): 130–138.

Tomchek SD, Dunn W (2007). Sensory processing in children with and without autism: A comparative study using the short sensory profile. *American Journal of Occupational Therapy* **61**(2): 190–200.

Tong VM, Huang CW, McIntyre T (2006). Promoting a positive cross-cultural identity: Reaching immigrant students. *Reclaiming Children & Youth* **14**(4): 203–208.

Towle A, Bainbridge L, Godolphin W, Katz A, Kline C, Lown B, *et al.* (2010). Active patient involvement in the education of health professionals. *Medical Education* **44**(1): 64–74.

Trevarthen C (1979). Communication and cooperation in early infancy: A description of primary intersubjectivity. *Before Speech: The Beginning of Interpersonal Communication*: 321–347.

Trevarthen C (2000). Musicality and the intrinsic motive pulse: Evidence from human psychobiology and infant communication. *Musicae Scientiae* **3**(1 suppl): 155–215.

Tyler TR, Lind AE, Hou AY (2000). Cultural values and authority relations: The psychology of conflict across cultures. *Psychology, Public Policy and Law* **6**(4): 1138–1163.

Verderber S (2010). *Innovations in Hospital Architecture*. Routledge.

Veselinova C (2014). Influencing communication and interaction in dementia. *Nursing & Residential Care* **16**(3): 162–166.

Volker DL, Kahn D, Penticuff JH (2004). Patient control and end-of-life care Part I: The advanced practice nurse perspective. *Oncology Nursing Forum* **31**(5): 945–953.

Vrij A, Pannell H, Ost J (2005). The influence of social pressure and black clothing on crime judgements. *Psychology, Crime & Law* **11**(3): 265–274.

Watzlawick P (1978). Intentionality and communication. *Journal of Communication* **28**(4).

Watzlawick P, Jackson DD (2010). On human communication (1964). *Journal of Systemic Therapies* **29**(2): 53–68.

Weber H, Stöckli M, Nübling M, Langewitz W (2007). Communication during ward rounds in internal medicine: An analysis of patient–nurse–physician interactions using RIAS. *Patient Education and Counseling* **67**(3): 343–348.

Weeks J, Hoare J (1979). Designing and living in a hospital: An enormous house. *Journal of the Royal Society of Arts*: 464–480.

Weiss PR (2000). Emotion and learning. *Training & Development* **54**(11): 44–48.

Wermke K, Leising D, Stellzig-Eisenhauer A (2007). Relation of melody complexity in infants' cries to language outcome in the second year of life: A longitudinal study. *Clinical Linguistics and Phonetics* **21**(11–12): 961–973.

Wilkinson G, Miers M (1999). *Power and Nursing Practice*. Palgrave Macmillan: London.

Willis Jr FN, Hamm HK (1980). The use of interpersonal touch in securing compliance. *Journal of Nonverbal Behavior* **5**(1): 49–55.

Windley D, Chapman M (2010). Support workers within learning/intellectual disability services perception of their role, training and support needs. *British Journal of Learning Disabilities* **38**(4): 310–318.

Wittgenstein L (1967). *Philosophical Investigations*. Oxford University Press: Oxford.

Woogara J (2005). Patients' rights to privacy and dignity in the NHS. *Nursing Standard* **19**(18): 33–37.

Wrong (1979). *Power: Its Forms, Bases and Uses*. Blackwell Publishing: Oxford.

Yip M-P (2012). A health literacy model for limited English speaking populations: Sources, context, process, and outcomes. *Contemporary Nurse: A Journal for the Australian Nursing Profession* **40**(2): 160–168.

Zeedyk S., Caldwell P., C. D (2009). How rapidly does Intensive Interaction promote social engagement for adults with profound learning disabilities? *European Journal of Special Needs Education* **24**(2): 119–137.

Zeedyk S. M., Davies C., Parry S., P. C (2009). Fostering social engagement in Romanian children with communicative impairments: The experiences of newly trained practitioners of Intensive Interaction. *British Journal of Learning Disabilities* **37**(3): 186–196.

Ziviani J, Lennox N, Allison H, Lyons M, Del Mar C (2004). Meeting in the middle: Improving communication in primary health care consultations with people with an intellectual disability. *Journal of Intellectual & Developmental Disability* **29**(3): 211–225.

INDEX